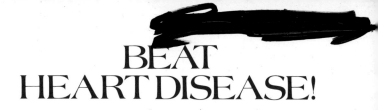

BEAT HEART DISEASE!

Dr Risteárd Mulcahy is a physician in Dublin who has devoted much of his professional work to the prevention of heart disease. He was the founder and President of the Irish Heart Foundation, is currently Chairman of the Foundation's research and information committee and is head of the Heart Disease Research Unit at St Vincent's Hospital, Dublin. He and his colleagues have published more than 100 scientific papers and books, mostly on the prevention of heart disease. Dr Mulcahy is a Past President of the Irish Medical Association.

Practising what he preaches, Dr Mulcahy exercises regularly, jog/walking around Dublin where he lives, practising calisthenics and playing tennis enthusiastically.

D1189256

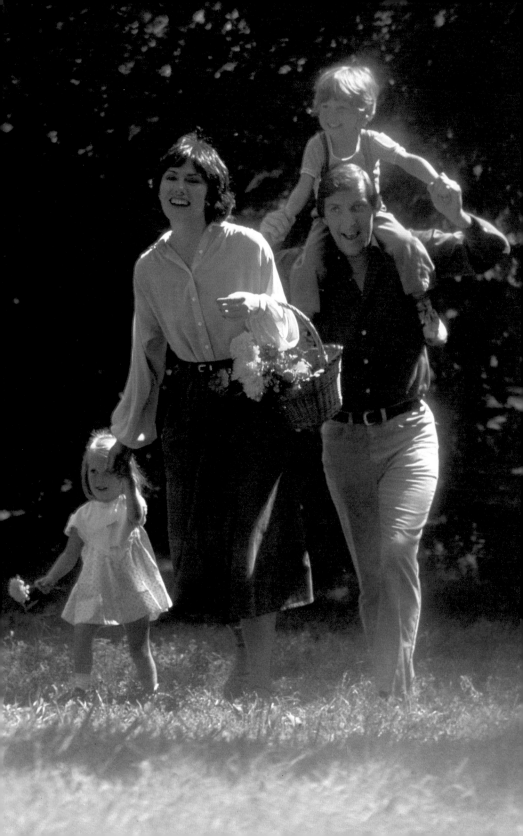

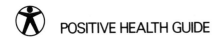 POSITIVE HEALTH GUIDE

BEAT HEART DISEASE!
A cardiologist explains how
you can help your heart and enjoy a
healthier life.

Risteárd Mulcahy
MD, FRCP, FRCPI

Foreword by Professor John Goodwin, MD, FRCP, FACC
President of the International Society
and Federation of Cardiology

MARTIN DUNITZ

© **Dr Risteárd Mulcahy** 1979
Second edition 1980

First published in the United Kingdom in 1979
by Martin Dunitz Limited, 12 Queensborough
Mews, Porchester Terrace, London W2 3AG

ISBN paperback 0 906348 05 6
ISBN hardback   0 906348 04 8

Studio photographs by Bill Ling
Location photographs by Simon Farrell

Text filmset by Inforum Ltd, Portsmouth

**British Library Cataloguing in Publication
Data**
Mulcahy, Risteárd
   Beat Heart Disease!
   – (Positive health guides)
   1. Heart – Diseases – Pevention
   I. Title   II Series
   616.1′2′05   RC682
   ISBN 0–906348–04–8
   ISBN 0–906348–05–6 Pbk.

Printed in Hong Kong
by South China Printing Co.

CONTENTS

For Richard, David, Hugh, Tina, Barbara and Lisa

FOREWORD

Professor J.F. Goodwin MD, FRCP, FACC
Professor of Clinical Cardiology
at the Royal Postgraduate Medical School, London
and President of the International Society and Federation of Cardiology

Dr Risteárd Mulcahy has devoted many years of his professional life to the study of the prevention of coronary heart disease. He has always been interested in health education and his enthusiasm as first President of the Irish Heart Foundation did much to advance research into heart disease in Ireland.

Beat Heart Disease! is his second book for the general public. In it he discusses the causes of, and practical methods for the prevention of coronary heart disease and stroke, explaining the basic pathological and physiological disorders in clear terms that are readily understandable.

Like all enthusiasts Dr Mulcahy emphasizes his views with vigour and in chapter two he points out, in no uncertain terms, the importance to good health of the better life; he also shows that illness can be caused by mistakes we can all too easily make in our daily lives. Exercise, Dr Mulcahy believes, is a key to health and he gives useful practical hints on how to keep fit. He also discusses diet and the problems caused by alcohol, cigarette smoking and high blood pressure, giving sensible comments on these important related aspects of coronary heart disease and stroke.

The book is not only useful, it is heartening and refreshing. Here is no miserable defeatist attitude or nihilism, but rather a positive, optimistic, cheerful approach, a beacon to all who may suffer from coronary heart disease and doubt that anything they or anyone else can do will help them.

The encouragement given in the book is reinforced by the sensible explanations and by the forceful style of the author. Dr Mulcahy writes as he speaks, with energy, clarity and humour; he cannot fail to inspire his readers.

As President of the International Society and Federation of Cardiology, an organization with the combined aims of research and education of physicians and the general public in the problems of heart disease, I welcome Dr Mulcahy's book and wish it the success that it deserves.

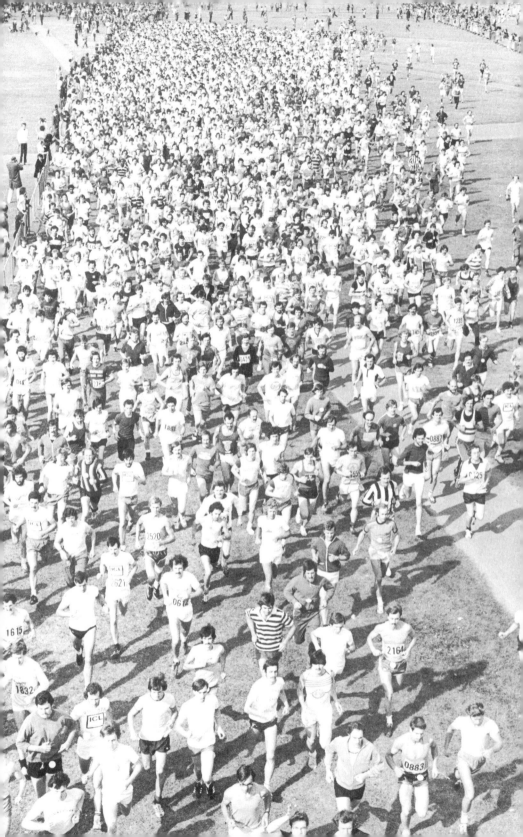

INTRODUCTION

Heart disease and stroke are the two most important causes of serious illness and premature death in Western society. The aim of this book is to help you reduce your chances of suffering heart disease or stroke, and to advocate a way of life that will combine health, longevity and happiness.

We start by looking at how the heart works and what causes angina, heart attack and stroke. An understanding of the causes of heart disease and the intelligent application of preventive measures could, I believe, lead to the virtual elimination of heart disease and stroke, at least for people under sixty-five or seventy years old.

Major factors in the present epidemic of heart disease are explored. These include lack of exercise, an unbalanced diet, cigarette smoking, excessive alcohol consumption and high stress levels. Advice on how to overcome these factors, if followed, could also help to eliminate many other non-cardiac conditions and play a major role in reducing psychiatric illness and premature ageing.

It is obvious that most people in our society do not anticipate illness, no matter how much they may neglect themselves and their health. If they become ill they confidently assume that doctors and medical science will come to their rescue. Yet we know that few of our contemporary chronic diseases can be cured and in most cases we can only expect temporary alleviation through drugs and surgery.

Instead of relying on drugs or surgery to maintain a healthy community, we should adopt more natural means to restore and maintain good health. The benefits of exercise, a natural diet, creative and active occupation and, most of all, knowledge based on good psychological, social and medical insights, are all-important if we are to create a disease-free world.

I believe that all the common illnesses of our time are due to the environment in which we live and to our adaptation to it. Pavlov, the great Russian physiologist, defined health as a state of being in equilibrium with surrounding nature. I believe that if you adapt your habits and behaviour to your environment you are assured of a healthier, longer and better life. This is what this book is all about.

If you have already suffered from a heart attack or stroke you can also benefit by appropriate life-style changes. Furthermore, if you adopt a better way of life you may well be healthier and happier after your illness than before.

LEFT: Marathon runs such as this are non-competitive and carefully graded. Physical fitness can help prevent heart disease and bring much happiness.

1 GOOD HEALTH AND A BETTER LIFE

Begin by looking at the way you regard your own health. Many people think it is the doctor's job to keep them healthy. But look at it another way and it becomes obvious that we all need to become active participants in maintaining our own good health. This responsible approach is particularly feasible in the prevention of heart disease and stroke – the two great killers of modern times – since their causes are predictable and largely preventable.

Most of the great epidemic diseases of the past have been overcome by social and cultural changes and by public preventive measures, rather than through the direct application of medical knowledge. This is true of cholera, tuberculosis, poliomyelitis and most of the infectious diseases. It could also be true of heart disease and stroke.

If you have had a heart attack or a stroke medical science can help to patch you up, but the contribution from physicians and surgeons is trivial compared to the contribution which could be made by adopting a more healthy way of life.

Some people, including doctors, are still sceptical that a particular way of life can influence the present epidemic of coronary disease and stroke. In this context it is worth looking at the statistics for heart disease and stroke in Western society and noting the changes that are taking place. These show that a fall in the frequency of heart disease and stroke in certain countries can be largely attributed to life-style changes brought about by public-health education and by individuals acting for their own good.

The pattern of heart disease

More than 80 per cent of adult heart disease in Western countries is caused by an obstructive disease of the coronary arteries called atherosclerosis. This silting-up process is explained in chapter three. The chart on page 25 shows the mortality from the disease in a number of countries and for both sexes for the years 1971-4. In many countries, coronary disease causes as much as 30 per cent of all deaths; in men during their active years (under sixty years) it causes 40 per cent or more deaths.

About 15 per cent of all deaths are caused by stroke. This condition is equally common in men and women and, after coronary disease and cancer, it is the third greatest killer in modern society.

For every 100 deaths from coronary attack there are about 150 survivors of an attack. These patients are contributing to the explosive increase in health-care costs, particularly in regard to the development of costly and complex diagnostic and treatment techniques. They are also a loss to the work force and to the economy, and place a serious emotional and social burden on themselves and their families.

Coronary disease, like stroke, leads to disability, loss of employment, social upheaval, human unhappiness and, at times, human despair.

There are now hopeful signs from countries like the United States and Finland that a more positive preventive approach is being taken by doctors and the public.

What is happening in the United States?

The frequency of coronary heart disease in the United States has fallen by about 20 per cent over the past eight years. This represents a dramatic reduction in deaths by as many as 116,000 per year and the fall is associated with a substantial reduction in stroke and a corresponding reduction in total mortality.

We now know that this improvement is not shared equally by the entire American population. It is more obvious among educated Americans, that is, college graduates, business executives and professional people.

The fall in the frequency of coronary heart disease and stroke reflects important life-style changes: these include changes in diet with a falling consumption of cholesterol-rich and saturated-fat foods, such as fat meat and dairy foods, and a rising consumption of polyunsaturated-fat foods, like vegetable oils and soft margarines. This change in diet is associated with a small but significant fall in national blood cholesterol levels.

Cigarette smoking is also considerably less according to Federal government statistics and, in addition, American physicians over the past ten years or so have been identifying and treating high blood pressure more efficiently than formerly. An enormous rise in the sale of running shoes and bicycles, to take two examples, demonstrates an increased interest in exercise.

Thus educated people in the United States are receptive to health education as provided by the American Heart Association, the American Cancer Society, the Department of Health, Education and Welfare and other agencies. They are responding in a positive way to health advice and if this trend continues there will be a dramatic reduction in coronary heart disease and stroke, and indeed in most of the common chronic diseases in this section of American society. This change in habits and life-style will, over a period of time, probably be reflected in American society as a whole.

The evidence currently available to us strongly suggests that changing smoking, diet and exercise habits and better control of high blood pressure are major factors influencing the improved health and life expectation of the American people. In my view developments in medical and surgical treatment over the past fifteen years have contributed in only a small way to this improved life expectation.

Does health education help?

Heart foundations and other agencies have played a major role in encouraging a healthier life through health education. These organizations are promoting the association of doctors and medical scientists with the community, and are dedicated to the control and elimination of the common chronic diseases in our society. The close contact of lay people with doctors in this way has been a major factor in breaking down the barriers between the medical profession and the public. As a result doctors have also become involved in the prevention of disease. The following case history demonstrates one way in which this can be done.

J.D. is a successful insurance salesman, aged fifty-one. Up to five years ago he led a completely sedentary life and was about 50 lb (23 kg) above his ideal weight. He was a big eater although sparing about drink. His blood fats were raised and abnormal, and his blood pressure was also persistently raised. He smoked heavily.

He saw a doctor about five years ago because of chronic low-back pain. A diagnosis of arthritis and disc trouble was made. He also complained of frequent fatigue, particularly after his day's work, and he complained of occasional boredom bordering on depression.

J.D. had no evidence of heart trouble at the time but he was obviously at very high risk for heart disease. Important life-style changes were proposed by his doctor. These included regular and active exercise, simple dietary changes and complete prohibition of smoking. He responded to this programme in a most enthusiastic and diligent manner.

He is now an entirely different person. He has lost 40 lb (18 kg) and has done so painlessly through his physical exercise programme and diet. He stopped smoking immediately but continues to take an occasional drink. The back trouble has long since vanished thanks to physical fitness and to weight control. His blood pressure and blood fats are normal. He is now at low risk for coronary disease and stroke, and no longer complains of fatigue or boredom. He spent three weeks last summer in France on a cycling vacation with his family. He described the holiday as the best he has ever had. The transition from a paunchy and inactive middle age to dynamic and youthful vigour is as much a source of surprise to his friends as it is a source of satisfaction to himself and his family.

J.D.'s case history above shows how further trouble was prevented. This primary prevention, as it is commonly called, aims to eliminate risk factors (such as smoking), encourage the taking of exercise and the control of harmful conditions such as high blood pressure. This is the most crucial part of long-term prevention and healthy living.

In my opinion, every penny spent on public education by a heart foundation is, in terms of health, happiness and productivity, worth thousands more than the vast sums spent on hospital services. Every one of us can put into practice this knowledge about the prevention of heart disease.

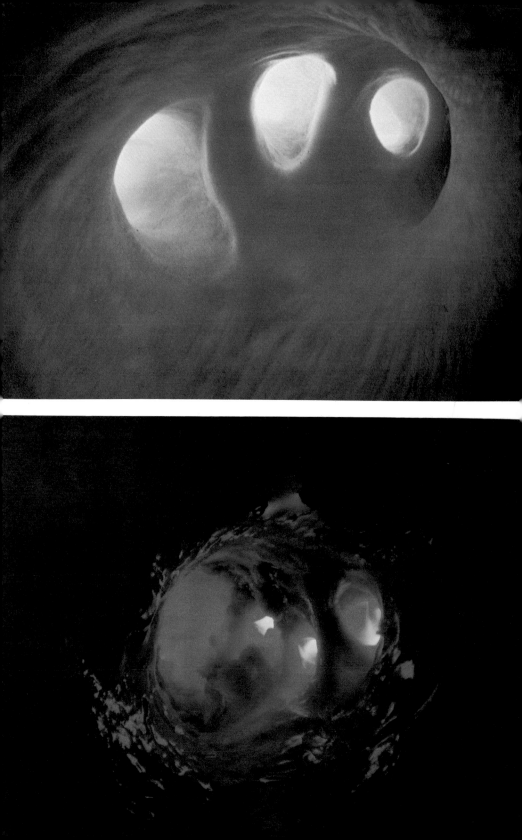

2 HOW THE HEART AND ARTERIES WORK

The heart

The heart is a twin pump, about the size of a clenched fist, and is functionally divided into two portions or sides. The right side of the heart receives blood from the main veins of the body and pumps the blood into the lungs. The left side receives the blood returning from the lungs and pumps it out through the arteries to all parts of the body (see below).

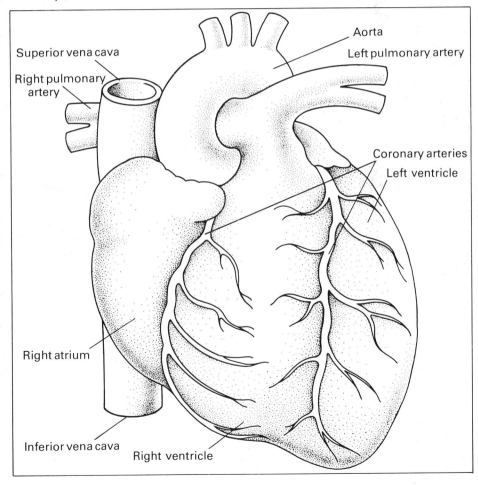

Superior vena cava
Right pulmonary artery
Aorta
Left pulmonary artery
Coronary arteries
Left ventricle
Right atrium
Inferior vena cava
Right ventricle

LEFT, ABOVE: Clear arteries of a one-year-old.
BELOW: Arteries of a sixty-year-old, silted up by atherosclerosis.

The flow of blood maintained by the heart is called the circulation. The blood returning to the right side of the heart lacks oxygen and contains waste products such as carbon dioxide. This is called venous blood and when it reaches the lungs through the right ventricle of the heart it gives up carbon dioxide and acquires fresh oxygen. This oxygen-rich blood is then re-circulated to all parts of the body through the left ventricle of the heart and the artéries (page 18).

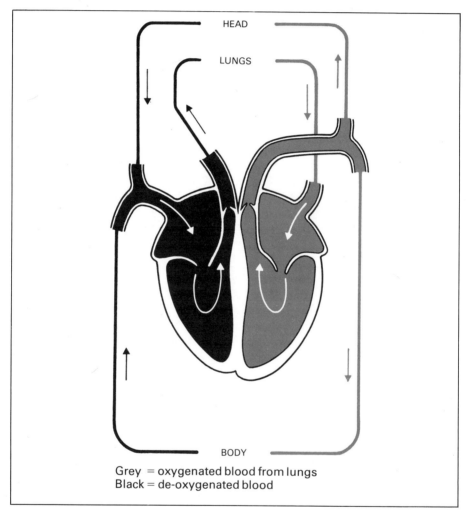

The circulation of blood from the body through the heart to the lungs; from the lungs the oxygenated blood returns to the heart and circulates to the rest of the body.

Oxygen is collected by the blood from the lungs, which are fine spongy organs made up of millions of tiny microscopic air sacs, or alveoli. These alveoli allow the oxygen-rich air to give up its oxygen to the arterial blood and to extract the waste carbon dioxide and other products from the venous blood.

The heart itself is made up of two essential components: the heart muscle and the valves. There are two valves on each side of the heart and they are strategically placed to ensure that the circulation of blood is maintained in the correct direction. Damage to the valves will interfere with the efficient pumping of the heart and valve disease is a common cause of heart failure and other complications.

Each side of the heart is made up of two chambers: the atrium and the ventricle. The atrium receives the blood returning to its side and allows it to flow into the ventricle during the period of relaxation, called diastole. The ventricle is the more powerful chamber and is the pumping portion which empties the blood into the main blood vessel. The atrium is protected by a valve (the tricuspid valve on the right side and the mitral valve on the left side) so that blood from the ventricle cannot be pumped back into it. The ventricle is protected by a valve at its exit (the pulmonary valve on the right side and the aortic valve on the left side) so that blood pumped into the vessels cannot return. The proper functioning of these valves is essential for effective blood circulation.

The heart muscle provides the pumping mechanism essential for maintaining the circulation. The amount of muscle in each chamber depends on the chamber's function and, because the left ventricle has the greatest amount of work to do in maintaining circulation to all parts of the body except the lungs, its muscle is thickest and most powerful.

Heart muscle is extraordinarily stable, adaptable and resilient, but its efficiency is entirely dependent on its supply of oxygen and nutrient-rich blood from the coronary arteries. If the heart muscle is deprived of oxygen it will cease to function in a matter of a minute or two, a condition which may lead to serious complications or to complete stoppage of the heart.

The arteries

The channels which carry the blood from the left side of the heart to the tissues of the body are called the arteries. From the main artery of the body, or aorta, the arteries branch continuously and diminish gradually in size until the blood eventually reaches the tiny microscopic capillaries. Here oxygen and nutrients are released and waste products are collected, while the blood continues to flow through to the veins and eventually to the right side of the heart (page 20).

Arteries are flexible, elastic, and strong tubes which, when healthy, can stand up to very considerable pressures. They are made up of three coats or layers, called the intima, media and adventitia.

The inner lining of the arteries or intima is very thin and very smooth, so that the flow of blood is not impeded in any way. This smooth lining is also essential to prevent blood from clotting. It is damage to, and thickening of, this smooth lining

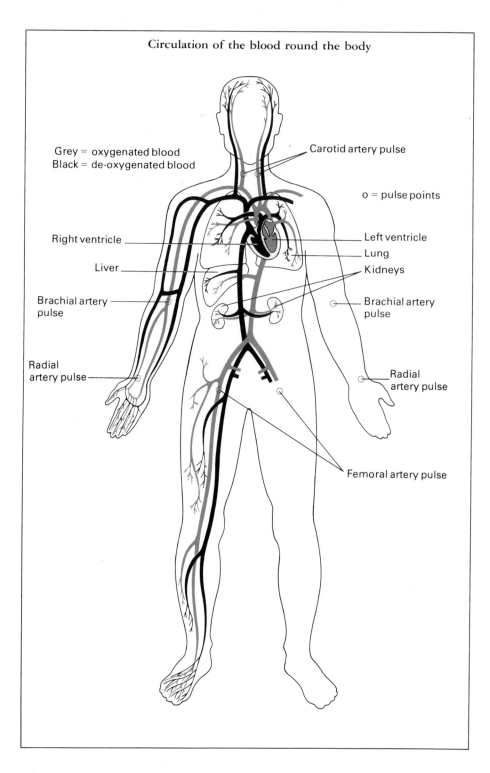

Circulation of the blood round the body

Grey = oxygenated blood
Black = de-oxygenated blood

Carotid artery pulse

o = pulse points

Right ventricle

Left ventricle

Lung

Liver

Kidneys

Brachial artery
pulse

Brachial artery
pulse

Radial
artery pulse

Radial
artery pulse

Femoral artery pulse

by a disease called atherosclerosis which causes coronary heart disease, stroke and other serious organic conditions. Atherosclerosis is discussed in chapter three.

The media or middle coat is thick and contains both muscle and elastic tissue. This layer gives the artery its strength and an ability to change the pressure or the distribution of blood-flow by contracting or relaxing. Over-activity of the media of the small arteries may be an important factor in causing high blood pressure.

The adventitia is a loose outer coat conveying nerves and tiny blood vessels to the medial coat. It also has an important function in attaching the blood vessels to the surrounding tissues and in protecting the arteries from infection.

Blockage of the coronary arteries, with consequent interference with heart muscle nutrition and function, is by far the commonest cause of heart disease today. It is generally caused by atherosclerosis.

Coronary arteries

There are two coronary arteries which arise from the main artery of the body, or aorta, just beyond the exit valve of the left ventricle. Called the right and left coronary arteries, they encircle the base of the heart like a crown and it is from this that the word coronary is derived (page 17). They send out large branches around the surface of the heart and these branches send numerous smaller branches deep into the heart muscle to provide a rich and continuous source of fresh arterial blood.

These two coronary arteries and their branches are prone to blockage from atherosclerosis. When these blockages are severe or numerous they may seriously affect the nutrition of the heart muscle and particularly the thick muscle of the left ventricle.

The pulse

Under resting conditions the left ventricle of the heart pumps about one fluid ounce (seventy cubic centimetres) of blood into the main artery with each heart beat. This influx of blood causes the elastic main artery to swell and this impulse is propelled along the vessel walls right to the end of the arterial system. This wave can be felt as a sudden impulse over the artery just after each heart beat. This pulse is traditionally felt by doctors and nurses in the radial artery at the wrist where the artery is close to the skin and is easily felt against the bone (called the radius). The pulse may be felt in many other places in the body and these locations are shown on page 20. You can easily identify your own pulse in these areas by checking with the diagram.

Blood pressure

Another important measurement is blood pressure. It is the pressure in the arterial system which ensures that blood will effectively reach all the tissues of the body in adequate amounts. See chapter ten for more details about blood pressure.

LEFT: The arteries carry the blood from the left ventricle to the tissues of the body and the veins return the blood to the right side of the heart and lungs.

3 WHAT CAN GO WRONG?

The silting-up of the arteries

When the arteries get silted-up over the years, the process is known as atherosclerosis, sometimes mistakenly called 'hardening of the arteries'. It starts in the intima or inner lining as small, flat yellow patches or streaks. These patches enlarge gradually, projecting into the arteries where they eventually cause serious interference with, or even total obstruction of, blood flow. The enlarged patches are called plaques. The process is usually a slow and gradual one, taking place over a period of years.

Initially the flat streaks contain pure cholesterol. This is a fatty substance normally present in the blood, but which is often excessive in people with atherosclerosis (pages 84–7). As the plaques enlarge, other substances appear and eventually the plaques may show the effects of degeneration, inflammation and haemorrhage or bleeding. When the plaque is big it may contain rather soft or porridge-like material. Hence the name 'atherosclerosis', derived from the Greek word for porridge.

When the plaque reaches an advanced stage, various complications may occur. It can become fragmented so that pieces dislodge and are carried further along the artery to cause obstruction. Such a fragment is called an embolus. The surface of the plaque may break down and form a raw area where a clot may develop. Clotting is common and will invariably cause a further reduction in blood flow. It may even cause a complete obstruction. This clotting is called a thrombosis, and is an important cause of an acute heart attack or stroke if there is underlying atherosclerosis.

Bleeding may also occur into the plaque, causing it to enlarge suddenly and leading to further obstruction of the artery.

The complications which arise from narrowing, obstruction, clotting and embolism lead to all the serious forms of heart disease and stroke so common in Western society today and may have sudden and dramatic effects. The symptoms, however, may be much less dramatic, perhaps appearing only from time to time when an increased blood supply is necessary during exercise or during other periods of increased oxygen demand. You may possibly have fairly advanced atherosclerosis without suffering any symptoms or complications because the atherosclerotic plaques have not yet reached a critical stage of development.

The cause of atherosclerosis

An enormous volume of research, particularly over the past thirty years, has established the most important causes of atherosclerosis. This research has been conducted by scientists in the laboratory, by doctors at the bedside, by research workers studying the distribution of disease in the community, and by surgeons and pathologists examining affected tissues during life or after death. We now know that atherosclerosis is associated with a number of common habits or characteristics in the individual.

The three most important of these are cigarette smoking, high blood pressure and abnormal blood fats. Other associated factors are stress, a family history of heart disease, lack of exercise and being a member of the male sex. Some relatively less common medical conditions, such as diabetes and underactivity of the thyroid gland, are also known to be associated with the atherosclerotic diseases. The charts on pages 85, 86 and 112 show how the risk factors of high blood pressure and high cholesterol affect the frequency of coronary disease. People who smoke, have high blood pressure and high cholesterol are twenty to thirty times more prone to heart attack than those who do not.

Which are the vulnerable arteries?

While atherosclerosis may occur in any artery of your body it has a notorious tendency to appear in certain important and vulnerable areas. The coronary arteries supplying the heart, the big arteries in the neck supplying the brain, the main artery of the body, or aorta, and its branches to the kidneys, intestines and legs, are particularly vulnerable. Obstruction in the coronary and neck arteries leads to coronary disease and stroke.

Plaque has a tendency to appear in areas of unusual hydraulic stress in the arteries. The word 'hydraulic' refers to the behaviour of liquids and, just as rough turbulent flood water will damage the banks of a river, so abnormal blood flow and pressures can damage the walls of an artery. These areas are often close to the origin of large arteries and one major obstruction over a short length of the artery may be the main cause of symptoms. Knowledge of the distribution of atherosclerotic plaques in certain arteries and of the influence of physical and hydraulic factors is of importance to your doctor in understanding the disease, in assisting exact diagnosis and in deciding on treatment methods.

How can we prevent atherosclerosis?

Doctors are now in the fortunate position of being able to help prevent coronary heart disease and stroke. Studying the habits or life-style of a population enables us to predict with accuracy that population's tendency to heart disease or stroke. Similarly, from studying your way of life and risk profile, a doctor can estimate the likelihood of you suffering heart disease or stroke. For instance, we can now study your smoking habits, blood-fat and blood-pressure levels and your degree of overweight and, by referring to risk-factor tables, make a fairly accurate estimate of your risk of future heart attack or stroke. This might sound cold and clinical but, if you are at high risk, you should be aware of this.

For example, we know that in two apparently healthy men of forty, where one smokes two packs of cigarettes a day, the smoker has about four times the risk of coronary attack and twice the risk of dying during the subsequent twenty years compared to the non-smoker. Other things being equal, the level of blood pressure and the level of cholesterol will also allow us to estimate risk of serious illness or premature death, as caused by a coronary heart attack. In fact, as an extreme but not particularly rare example, a forty-year-old smoker of two packs a day who has high cholesterol and high blood pressure has thirty times or more the risk of getting a coronary attack during the subsequent twenty years compared to a non-smoker of the same age with normal cholesterol and blood pressure. We are talking now about the *risk* of having a heart attack; this is a risk not an inevitability.

Research shows that stopping smoking and treating high blood pressure will reduce the risk of heart attack and stroke. If you are overweight your health will improve if you lose weight and alter your diet to take in less animal fats. An important function of the medical profession today, and the main objective of this book, is to provide guidance on life-style changes which will eliminate the athero-sclerotic diseases without in any way leading to undesirable or inacceptable changes in the modern way of life.

Coronary heart disease

Atherosclerotic disease of the coronary arteries may occur in a variety of ways, depending on the extent, number and condition of the atherosclerotic plaques.

First, the disease may be without symptoms and be suspected only by inference because of a high-risk profile. Such cases may be more precisely identified by doing a maximum exercise or stress electrocardiogram. The electrocardiogram (ECG – see page 31) will be normal at rest but early changes of a reduced blood supply will be shown by the test during, and immediately after, strenuous exertion.

A special X-ray of the coronary arteries (coronary arteriogram) will show obstruc-tions, but the complexity of this technique makes it undesirable for all except those with advanced cases of heart disease who may need surgery.

The disease in the coronary arteries may be insufficient to cause total obstruction but may limit the increased flow needed by the heart muscle when more oxygen is required, such as during exercise. On these occasions the limited blood circulation will lead to a temporary state of lack of oxygen or ischaemia, which you will feel immediately as an unpleasant tightness or pain in the chest. The condition is called angina pectoris or angina of effort.

If there is a sudden obstruction in a coronary artery, caused by a fresh clot or by bleeding into a plaque or the dislodgement of a plaque, the heart muscle beyond the obstruction may be totally deprived of its blood supply. This sudden event is usually heralded by prolonged pain and is called a myocardial infarction (myocardial: heart muscle; infarction: destruction of tissue) or, in older medical terminology, a coronary thrombosis or occlusion. This is the most common form of heart attack.

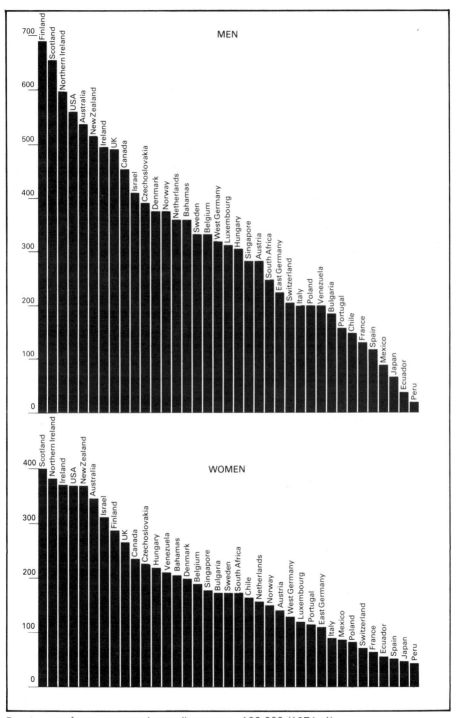

Death rates from coronary heart disease per 100,000 (1971–4)

Angina

What are the causes?

Angina or angina pectoris, translated from the Latin, means chest pain. Angina is often called angina of effort because the chest discomfort which you may feel is usually brought on by exercise or by some other factor which increases the oxygen needs of the heart.

By far the most common cause of angina is atherosclerosis of the coronary arteries. Other rare causes are damage to the exit valve of the left ventricle and anaemia or reduction in the oxygen-carrying capacity of the blood.

When the silting-up process is fairly advanced the arteries cannot accommodate the increased blood flow required when you exercise. The temporary shortage of oxygen-rich blood causes your heart muscle to go into an uncomfortable or painful cramp. This is the pain of angina.

A few people, particularly middle-aged women, may have the symptoms of angina without significant coronary disease. Rest assured you will suffer no ill-effects from this innocent condition, which a doctor can fairly easily recognize.

How does angina feel?

You may experience a tight feeling, oppression or pain in the centre of the chest behind the breastbone. This somtimes spreads into one or both arms, the neck, or jaw, through to the back (rarely in other directions). The pain is constant or continuous while it lasts and is never sharp, stabbing or of only a few seconds' duration. It may feel to you like indigestion. The pain generally occurs only on exertion – such as walking. You will probably find that the pain occurs every time you walk a certain distance or at a certain speed. It is relieved by stopping or even by slowing down, and when you start walking again you may be able to walk a good deal further than before. This improved capacity to walk after stopping is very common and is called 'second wind' angina.

Some things may aggravate angina, such as walking in cold, windy, blustery weather or after a heavy meal. Emotional upset or tension will have the same effect and excitement or emotional upset alone may be sufficient in themselves to cause angina. A tense television show or football match may bring on the pain. For some people, angina is more likely to occur at certain times of the day.

Walking is not the only exercise that brings on symptoms. Cycling or any other sustained exercise involving the use of the legs has the same effect. Arm movements, even when sustained and even when part of relatively heavy work, will not usually trouble you, but there are occasional exceptions to this rule.

Angina is commoner among men than women in middle age, but is equally common in both sexes in the older age groups.

What your doctor will be looking for

Once angina has been confirmed you will be fully examined before treatment is started. Examination will reveal the condition of the heart muscle and valves,

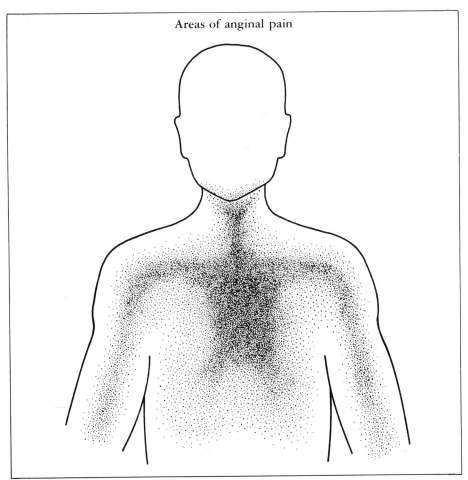

Areas of anginal pain

Anginal pain is felt most frequently high up in the centre of the chest but it often radiates to the shoulders, arms, neck and jaw.

whether there is evidence of trouble in arteries elsewhere in the body and whether important risk factors exist, such as high blood pressure and obesity. An examination will also help to identify any disease or disorders in other parts of your body.

Investigation may include a number of diagnostic tests. An electrocardiogram will reveal the presence of any heart-muscle damage and an exercise or stress electrocardiogram is invaluable in confirming the diagnosis of angina and in establishing the extent and severity of the atherosclerosis in the arteries. You may be asked to help with other simple tests which will identify important contributory factors to the underlying atherosclerosis. These factors include high blood pressure, diabetes and reduced function of the thyroid gland. A more sophisticated test includes a direct X-ray of the coronary arteries which will give detailed information about the extent and severity of the disease and the effects on the heart muscle and its function (see page 35).

27

Treatment of angina

Angina is only a symptom but it may restrict you, particularly in relation to your physical exercise, sport and work. To your doctor, who will be interested in your long-term well-being and life expectation, however, angina is of special significance. It indicates damage to the underlying arteries and therefore the risk of developing myocardial infarction or heart attack. Your doctor will therefore not only treat the pain but also attempt to slow down, stop or even reverse the atherosclerotic process in the arteries. The complications of angina are mentioned, not to cause anxiety but to encourage you to adopt a better life-style, to accept treatment and thus to improve your health and life expectation.

If you are suffering from angina you may develop nervous symptoms such as chest pains and giddiness because of your natural concern and anxiety about the illness and its significance. These symptoms include vague pains, aches and feelings of breathlessness and they can be disabling at times. They can be easily identified by an experienced physician and will often clear up completely in response to explanation and reassurance and after a return to normal work and exercise.

Risk factor control The most crucial part in the treatment of angina is the elimination of risk factors. Regular exercise, a return to a normal, active life, weight control and stopping smoking often improve or eliminate your painful symptoms. In a study at my own hospital we have shown that patients with coronary heart disease who stop smoking are less likely to develop further heart trouble and have a much improved life expectation. Lowering cholesterol may also be worthwhile and recent work suggests that lowering high blood pressure is also beneficial.

The elimination of risk factors must be permanent and for this reason a patient should return once or twice a year to his doctor to ensure that the secondary prevention programme is being carried out effectively. Doctors are only too familiar with the well-intentioned patient who co-operates enthusiastically after a life-threatening illness. He will be careful about cholesterol, blood pressure and weight control. He will stop smoking and will become physically fit and active, but so often, when he returns to normal health and pursuits and perhaps feels better than he has done for years, he will slowly drift back to his old habits, only to return eventually to the doctor with fresh coronary trouble. Because this is a fairly typical human response we all need to be aware of how easy it is to slip backwards. Nevertheless, prevention is always more satisfactory than cure.

The importance of physical fitness is illustrated by the case history of a man aged fifty-one who had suffered from angina of effort at the age of forty. He was a heavy smoker and overweight at that time. He gave up smoking, got his weight down to normal and became physically very active. His angina improved and he is able to do much more. He walks further and faster now.

This man is now lean and as physically active as any forty-year-old. He jog/walks and cycles a lot and he is entirely free from symptoms. He looks younger than his years and believes that his illness of eleven years ago has helped him to lead a more enjoyable, active and happier life.

28

Drugs have a part to play in the treatment of angina, either to relieve pain and thus increase exercise capacity, or to treat risk factors, such as high blood pressure. Drug treatment should not deflect us from focusing attention on the fundamental cause of angina: that is, atherosclerosis.

Efforts to ameliorate the atherosclerotic process will lead to fewer heart attacks and this should be the cornerstone of modern treatment. Most people who co-operate with treatment can look forward to many years of active and healthy life.

Surgery Coronary artery surgery is aimed at by-passing the obstructions in the coronary arteries by using strips of the patient's own leg veins or by grafting branches of the internal mammary artery. It has been increasingly practised for over ten years. The value of surgery remains undecided but it has been shown to be useful in relieving the pain of angina. Surgery is not advisable, however, without first trying other forms of medical treatment. Unfortunately, too often surgery is put forward as the treatment of choice before the effects of controlling the key risk factors, such as smoking, have been seen. Exercise programmes and pain-relieving drugs should also be tried first. If you have angina you will probably find that it is not disabling (requiring surgery) if you accept comprehensive medical treatment over a reasonable trial period. Too often the decision to operate is related more to the attitudes and views of the cardiologist and the heart surgeon than to the actual severity of the symptoms.

Apart from the treatment of angina, by-pass surgery may be used if you suffer from other coronary heart conditions. Coronary artery surgery can only be performed after careful investigation, including a coronary arteriogram, to identify the location, severity and number of obstructions which may require by-passing.

Live a healthy life

If you have angina you should avoid tension and stress in ordinary day-to-day affairs and should enjoy regular periods of leisure and relaxation. A rest period every day after lunch or on return from work, may be advised. Any emotional or psychological problems should be discussed with your doctor. Football matches, tense television programmes and other tension-causing situations are best avoided.

You may develop a more acute attack or myocardial infarction. Such an event is often preceded by warning symptoms. If these are immediately reported to your doctor he can reduce the risk of complications by advising a period of rest and observation at home or in a coronary care unit. You should report an increase in the frequency or severity of the anginal pain or if the pain begins to occur at rest, or if it fails to respond to pain-relieving drugs. Unusual and prolonged fatigue occurring for no obvious reason may also be a warning symptom. If the fatigue does not clear up within a day or two, and particularly after a short period of rest, it should be reported to your doctor.

Anginal pain often improves considerably or clears up completely if you follow advice about regular physical exercise and avoid obvious risks like smoking. In other people it may remain constant and non-progressive for years, without interfering with normal activity. This is nature's way of preventing you from overdoing things.

An optimistic view of your future health and longevity is usually justified if you follow medical advice and stick to a healthy way of life.

Acute heart attack

About 95 per cent of patients suffering from an acute heart attack or myocardial infarction have atherosclerosis of the coronary arteries. Various terms are commonly used by doctors and the general public to describe a heart attack. These include coronary thrombosis, coronary occlusion, myocardial infarction and acute coronary insufficiency. Some of these names lack precision from the scientific point of view and the two terms recommended (for their precise meaning) are acute coronary insufficiency and myocardial infarction. When a patient gets an acute coronary attack, he will have one of the above two conditions.

Acute coronary insufficiency is the least common form of attack. There is a sudden reduction in blood supply to part of the heart muscle because of temporary obstruction or spasm in the affected artery. The muscle cannot function properly and goes into a painful cramp. After some minutes or hours, however, the blood supply improves, the heart muscle begins to function again and the symptoms clear up completely.

Myocardial infarction implies the destruction of heart muscle and occurs in about 80 per cent of people who suffer an acute coronary attack. Here the blood supply is cut off completely to part of the heart muscle. Within a few hours the affected heart muscle dies and is no longer capable of assisting the pumping action of the heart. The gravity of the heart attack and the subsequent chance of making a full recovery largely depend on the amount of heart muscle that is damaged. If only a small part of the muscle is involved, as happens with many people, complications are unusual. Nearly all these patients make a full recovery with no subsequent impairment of heart muscle function.

When the heart muscle is deprived of its blood supply for more than an hour or two, the cells undergo permanent changes and the heart muscle undergoes destruction and degeneration. This is called an infarct in medical terminology and hence the term myocardial infarction. The dead muscle tissue is gradually removed by the body's healing process and very quickly healing and scar formation occurs. The speed of healing varies according to the extent of the damaged muscle. It is usually completed in six weeks although the healing area is perfectly secure before this.

The causes of a heart attack
It is seldom clear what causes an acute attack in the coronary-prone person. Often it is attributed to an accident, an emotional upset, excessive exercise or strain at work, plus a variety of other causes. In fact there is little evidence to show that heart attacks have a triggering-off mechanism. You may experience an attack at any time of the day or night, at home as well as at work, and in bed as well as when active. Only if you have had an operation or a serious injury (and are also coronary-prone) can your doctor anticipate a heart attack.

The symptoms of heart attack

By far the most common symptom is chest pain which is usually described as gripping, vice-like or tight, and is continuous for periods of up to some hours. The pain may feel like indigestion and is usually, but now always, most intense high up behind your breastbone. It may radiate from this position, notably into your arms, neck, jaw, back and occasionally down into the upper abdomen (page 27). You may also experience restlessness and cold sweating. During the acute stage of a heart attack you will almost certainly look very pale.

If, on the other hand, it is somebody else who is having a heart attack there are certain things you can do to help. Leave the person undisturbed and alert a doctor. If a doctor is not available contact the mobile coronary care service. If neither is available, drive the patient to the nearest hospital if he is not too bad. If you can do none of these avoid all unnecessary noise and excitement and allow the patient to rest until assistance arrives.

Tests for myocardial infarction

Examination by your doctor may confirm the suspicion of a heart attack. You will probably be asked to take simple tests to confirm the diagnosis beyond all doubt. These include an electrocardiogram (ECG) and enzyme tests.

The ECG records the minute electrical changes occurring in heart muscle cells. These electrical changes are constant in a healthy heart but they undergo a very well-recognized alteration with coronary insufficiency or infarction. The ECG provides information about the location, extent and severity of the infarction and about complications such as heart rhythm, heart rate and electrical conduction.

Enzyme tests help to confirm diagnosis since acutely damaged heart muscle cells quickly release chemical substances into the surrounding tissues and bloodstream. These substances are called enzymes and can be readily identified. Enzyme tests also give useful information about the timing and severity of the attack.

In certain, unusual cases, ECG and enzyme tests fail to give definite results and radio-active material is used to identify areas of myocardial infarction.

Other diagnostic tests may be employed in special cases and for special purposes, such as assessing the amount of damage to the heart muscle and estimating the degree of impairment of the pumping function of the heart. They may also be needed to check the electrical conduction system of the heart, a complicated electrical network like a telephone system which automatically controls the heart beat.

How is a heart attack treated?

If you have had a heart attack your treatment can be divided into two parts: short-term treatment of the acute attack, followed by long-term advice that you should follow. Treatment at the acute stage is usually based on anticipating, preventing and treating the various complications which occur in the early stages of the heart attack.

The greatest advance in treatment in recent years has been the development of the coronary care unit and the mobile care unit. In these units doctors can identify and treat the complications which may occur during the acute stage and which may be responsible for serious or even fatal consequences. In recent years we have learned a lot about the prevention and treatment of heart attack complications and these are described below.

Abnormal heart rhythms The normal heart beats regularly and steadily because of a built-in electrical controlling system. This electrical system is controlled by a special group of cells in the right atrium, called the sinoatrial node. This node acts as a pacemaker to control the rate of the heart and to ensure that the beats occur regularly.

During an acute attack the electrical system can be disturbed. This can lead to various changes of heart rate and rhythm, some of which are of no importance and require no treatment. Other changes have serious consequences, however, and may lead to total failure of the heart to contract in an orderly way, and therefore to sudden heart failure.

Thanks to our increasing knowledge of these disturbances, we are now able to anticipate them, and so prevent them; or we can stop them with appropriate treatment when they occur. The types of irregularities which can occur are too numerous to mention here, but their occurrence during the acute stage of a coronary attack provides one of the principal reasons for the development of the coronary care unit.

Heart failure This is the expression used to describe the failure of one or both ventricles to maintain an adequate circulation to the body. It is a form of gradual power failure, caused by a reduction in the force of the normal contraction of the ventricle.

Doctors can now recognize the early signs of power failure and, with appropriate treatment, prevent this complication in all patients except the minority who have very severe heart muscle damage.

Heart block When there is an interruption in the electrical conduction of the heart impulse, heart block occurs. It is a relatively common temporary condition during the acute stage and, if necessary, heart block can be treated by using a temporary artificial pacemaker.

What helps recovery?
Nearly all the important complications of an acute heart attack occur during the first day or two of the illness. Most of the skilled medical and nursing attention which the patient requires will be packed into these early days. Coronary ambulances and coronary care units provide this intensive care at the early stage.

Once the heart muscle damage is healed it is the exception rather than the rule to experience any complications. If you have had an acute heart attack, particularly if you are young, you can achieve a recovery which allows you to return to a normal active life. You may require some medical supervision afterwards, but you are unlikely to be restricted, or have to follow any exacting form of medical treatment.

Doctors are now taking a much less cautious approach to heart attack during the acute stage. It is usual to get a patient out of bed within a few days of admission to hospital and many people are active and well enough to go home within seven to ten days.

Active movements of the legs and arms and deep breaths are encouraged from the time of admission and, except in certain complicated cases, you will be encouraged to be increasingly active as soon as you get out of bed. You will find that exercises are beneficial because they reduce the risk of clotting in the veins and lungs during the acute stage, they keep your muscles in trim, and this helps your recovery. Exercises also help you to get better, in a subtle way, by showing that you are well on the way to recovery.

Getting back to a normal life
When you return home you should start an exercise and physical fitness programme (see pages 38–83). The type of exercise programme you choose will need to be tailored to your age, physical limitations, circumstances, inclinations and occupation. Such a programme must be organized as a long-term project and as part of your normal daily life. Doctors may differ about the type and degree of physical exercise which is needed after a heart attack, but professional opinion increasingly favours a gradual build-up to optimum physical fitness without excessively severe or competitive exertion.

Except in special circumstances there is no merit in leading a sedentary life. People who adopt a regular exercise programme and have a high level of physical fitness will benefit considerably. Apart from the obvious physical and psychological benefits of exercise, it may slowly improve the circulation to your heart muscle and will help in weight control, lowering of blood fat and in overcoming the smoking habit. Irrespective of your age and previous habits physical fitness can be attained through gradually increasing activity over a period of weeks or months. Avoid sudden exercise and let your doctor supervise your progress.

Patients often ask their doctor when they are being discharged about resuming normal activities such as driving the car, gardening, shovelling snow or indulging in sexual intercourse. Each case must, of course, be considered on its merits but, except in an unusually complicated case, people can return gradually to all normal activities. Doctors will seldom forbid a patient to drive a car, gardening is encouraged as one form of active exercise and sexual intercourse is seldom discouraged although it may be necessary to curb the patient's enthusiasm for the first week or two after discharge from hospital. Shovelling snow is a different matter and should only be allowed if it is part of a patient's normal physical activity and well within his physical prowess.

Most people should be fit to return to a normal active life within three to four weeks after discharge from hospital. From my experience, rapid and active rehabilitation and a return to a normal life are in no way harmful.

At my hospital in Dublin, among 282 patients under sixty years who left hospital following a coronary attack, 75 per cent were back at work within three months of the start of the illness and 93 per cent eventually returned to work. Apart from five patients who returned to lighter work, all returned to their previous occupations, irrespective of how heavy or responsible their work might have been. Of the twenty-two (7 per cent) patients who failed to return to work, only nine patients were invalided because of the direct effect of the heart attack.

Medical causes for failure to return to work are therefore not common, and even when such causes exist they are not always directly due to the heart illness. Very often, failure to return to normal arises from an excessively cautious attitude on the part of the patient's doctor or relatives.

You are generally advised to have a full check-up about three weeks after discharge from hospital. This enables the doctor to check progress and monitor treatment. It also provides an opportunity to plan long-term treatment.

It is not possible to predict the future health of any individual with coronary heart disease. In the same survey at my hospital, however, all the patients who had survived a coronary attack were monitored for a period of four years. The mortality over the four-year period was 13.6 per cent (thirty-four patients), being an average annual mortality of 3.4 per cent. The greatest mortality occured in the first year (fourteen deaths), after which the mortality dropped to an average annual figure of 2.5 per cent. it is obvious that the long-term outlook depends to some extent on the severity of the heart attack, but another notable influence on future health is the subsequent smoking habits of the patients.

In those who continued to smoke as heavily as before, the mortality rate was 29 per cent, while among those who reduced considerably, stopped, or who were non-smokers at the time of the attack, the mortality was only 11 per cent. Stopping smoking appears to be the most effective way to recovery in patients who have survived a coronary attack. I also believe that future research will show that control of high blood pressure, obesity and high cholesterol levels will also have a beneficial effect. An active and permanent exercise programme can also play an important role in controlling risk factors like a high cholesterol level, and in improving life expectation.

Claims that drugs and coronary artery surgery improve survival and reduce the number of further attacks have been made but the evidence for these claims is so far not convincing and we must await further research.

What is a stroke?

A stroke may occur in various ways and with various degrees of severity. It may be a temporary or permanent condition, depending on the location, extent and permanence of the brain damage.

The term is used when paralysis or other central nervous system disturbances are caused by interference with the blood supply to the brain. Such interference may be caused by rupture of a brain or cerebral artery, commonly associated with very high and poorly controlled blood pressure. It may also be caused by embolism, where a clot is carried from the heart or arteries to the brain, but it is caused most commonly by narrowing and obstruction of atherosclerotic arteries supplying the brain.

The commonest form of stroke is a weakness or paralysis of the face, arm, and leg on one side of the body due to obstruction of a cerebral artery on the opposite side. This artery supplies the nerve fibres to the affected muscles before the fibres cross over lower down in the brain.

How to recognize stroke

Very frequently, patients who develop a stroke may get warning symptoms, such as temporary weakness or unsteadiness of the limbs, unusual sensory disturbances such as one-sided pins and needles and numbness, transient disturbances of vision, fainting attacks and unusual headaches. These may or may not be followed by a fully developed stroke. You should take notice of these warning symptoms, which are referred to as transient ischaemic attacks and tell your doctor about them; you could save yourself from a stroke and resulting paralysis.

If somebody develops sudden weakness or paralysis of one limb or of one side, if there is obvious difficulty with speech or if collapse is followed by stupor or unconsciousness you should immediately contact a doctor or hospital. If the person is unconscious remove false teeth and pull the tongue forward so it doesn't interfere with breathing.

Your doctor will be looking for other signs of a susceptibility to stroke. The presence of badly controlled high blood pressure is a major risk factor and the presence of disease in the coronary arteries and elsewhere is a warning signal. An examination may help the doctor to identify atherosclerotic disease in the main vessels of the neck and in the eyes.

A number of useful diagnostic tests can establish the presence of plaques in the neck and cerebral arteries. These include an arteriogram where opaque substances are injected to allow accurate X-ray pictures of the inside of the arteries. Ultrasound techniques may also be used for the same purpose.

Can stroke be prevented?

A stroke is a tragic event in anybody's life. Apart from the immediate risk of death, the stroke victim may be left with permanent paralysis and speech disturbances which may prevent him from leading a normal life; he is often severely disabled and unable to look after himself. The treatment and rehabilitation of stroke patients have improved in recent years, but nevertheless stroke still causes widespread misery and disability. However, we do have powerful weapons with which we can reduce the frequency of this catastrophe.

The great majority of strokes are caused either by atherosclerosis or more especially by high blood pressure. Abnormal blood fats and cigarette smoking are also important causes. There has been a dramatic fall in the incidence of stroke in the United States over the past twenty years or more, partly because of the better identification and control of high blood pressure (see page 111). This improvement is also apparent to a lesser degree in other Western countries and I have little doubt that stroke could become a relative rarity, at least in people under sixty-five years, if there were proper control of high blood pressure, elimination of cigarette smoking and encouragement towards healthier eating and exercise habits.

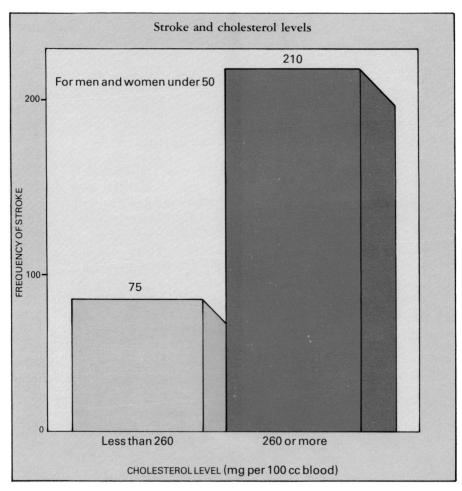

Stroke and cholesterol levels

For men and women under 50

FREQUENCY OF STROKE

200 –

100 –

0

210

75

Less than 260   260 or more

CHOLESTEROL LEVEL (mg per 100 cc blood)

In younger adults stroke is clearly related to the cholesterol level in the blood. The higher the cholesterol level the more likely a stroke.

The incidence of stroke in Ireland is similar to other Western countries. Fourteen per cent of all deaths and 10 per cent of deaths in people under sixty-five years were attributed to stroke in 1974. For every 100 persons of all age groups dying from the disease there were about 120 who survived three months or more. Of the survivors, nearly 75 per cent had some degree of paralysis or speech impairment one year later and 25 per cent were still bed-ridden.

The treatment of stroke

We can achieve some limited success in the treatment of the patient with stroke or threatened stroke. For the threatened stroke patient a by-pass operation of the arterial obstructions may be successful, particularly if combined with control of high blood pressure and other risk factors. Even without an operation, risk-factor control

36

may be successful. A by-pass operation is remedial at the most, not curative, and these operations do put an increased load on the community and health services. A rational society must give first priority to prevention.

The patient with an established stroke can be helped by modern methods of rehabilitation. In every centre of rehabilitation nowadays miracles of recovery can be witnessed in determined and well-motivated people. Some people may eventually return to their old occupations or may be successfully retrained for other work. Most recoveries from stroke are a tribute to the ingenuity and progress of modern medicine but are also a less obvious reflection of our failure to give proper priority to preventive medicine.

Your chances of a stroke are remote if you have not got uncontrolled high blood pressure, if you do not smoke cigarettes and if your weight, blood fat and blood sugar levels are normal.

Leg vessel disease

Atherosclerosis may also affect the arteries of the legs, kidneys and intestines; atherosclerosis of the legs is by far the most common and important of these in the active age groups.

Disease of the leg vessels is not unusual. There may be no symptoms initially but, as the obstruction in the arteries increases, you will begin to complain of pain in the calf muscles and, less often, in the thigh muscles and buttocks on the affected side when you walk. The cramp pain is not unlike the pain of angina and is caused by the same thing: that is, a deficient supply of oxygen-rich blood to the muscles during exercise. When you stop walking the pain will go fairly quickly only to return when you walk the same distance again.

This symptom is called intermittent claudication (claudicatio, Latin for lameness) and varies in intensity according to the degree of obstructive disease in the arteries. It may be so severe as to prevent you from walking more than fifty or 100 yards.

Increasing obstruction in the arteries, whether by worsening disease, clot formation or embolism, may mean that the blood doesn't circulate properly. This leads to serious nutritional problems and, eventually, to gangrene and loss of the limb.

No worthwhile drug or medical treatment is available but surgical treatment may help to by-pass obstruction or provide strips of new arteries. Surgical treatment can also improve the nutrition of the affected limb, although it cannot cure the disease in the arteries.

Leg vessel disease is associated with the same risk factors as coronary and cerebral disease, but is particularly associated with cigarette smoking. It is rare in non-smokers and almost unknown in non-smokers under sixty years. If you have this disease and stop smoking it is unlikely to get worse. The pain on walking often gets better and may clear up completely.

Many people who are severely limited by claudication can walk long distances without symptoms when they stop smoking and take up a graduated walking or exercise programme.

4 EXERCISE–
THE KEY TO HEALTH

The quality of life is greatly improved by physical exercise, hobbies and sport. The importance of leisure time in general, and physical exercise in particular, is greatest for the person who has a job that provides little opportunity for either exercise or variety.

How exercise can help

Exercise in its many forms is the best way of counteracting the stresses associated with overcrowding and city living and is not concerned solely with the achievement of physical fitness. It also encourages a greater respect for our bodies and is a way of improving our mental adaptation to the stresses of modern life. It is a healthy substitute for less worthy activities such as drinking, smoking and eating to excess. People who stop smoking, and eating or drinking excessively may be left with a void. In my experience alternatives are required. Exercise and sport are the easiest and healthiest alternatives.

The active, fit person is aware of the joy of movement and that enjoyment increases when the exercise is practised regularly and efficiently. In its various forms exercise also has important social implications. For instance, as a shared activity it strengthens family and group loyalties and improves social relations.

Physical and psychological benefits
Regular exercise and physical fitness will greatly reduce the frequency of the hypokinetic or sedentary diseases. These include obesity, arthritis, rheumatism, disc trouble, diabetes, high blood pressure, coronary disease, stroke and depression. While many of these conditions have multiple causes, they are much less likely to occur in the physically fit, either because physical fitness prevents or postpones the condition, as with arthritis and rheumatism, or the physically-fit person leads a life-style which protects from illness such as coronary disease and stroke.

I would like to emphasize the beneficial effects of exercise in combating depression and other psychiatric conditions such as chronic anxiety. Depressed and anxious people greatly benefit from regular physical exercise. Sadly, this approach is neglected by many psychiatrists, who are more committed to the use of drugs. Drugs are indispensable at times in the treatment of psychiatric illness but, in many instances, the track-suit is more effective than the tranquillizer.

If you suffer from depression, whatever its cause, and you can bring yourself to walk, jog or run a few miles a day, you will feel the better for it and you will be starting on the road to recovery. Lonely people will also benefit by following a regular exercise programme, not only through the contacts they may make while exercising but also because regular activity is fulfilling in itself.

Research by the Irish Heart Foundation shows how important exercise is in the prevention of coronary disease and stroke. The Foundation's research is based on a study of more than 15,000 adult males in the community. It shows that physical exercise does not necessarily protect directly against coronary disease and stroke, but the person who is active during his leisure time is less likely to smoke and over-eat, has lower blood pressure and blood cholesterol levels. The risk of atherosclerosis is consequently less. This almost certainly accounts for the smaller number of heart attacks among physically active people, because exercise reduces high cholesterol and high blood pressure levels, and contributes fundamentally to weight control. See also the report of the Framingham group (page 87).

Last, but not least, physical exercise postpones old age, although it does not necessarily increase longevity. If you exercise you will retain a youthful appearance and figure and you are less liable to develop the effects of age – the bent back, limited neck movements, reduced joint mobility and thinning muscles. Moreover, you are less liable to the increasing depression and sense of isolation of old age, and to all the sedentary diseases which we mistakenly believe to go hand in glove with old age.

All the tissues of the body were designed for use, especially the muscles, joints, sinews and bones – the tissues which make up the musculoskeletal system. Disuse of these tissues leads to wasting and to loss of strength, stamina and efficiency, finally to loss of function and to degenerative changes such as arthritis and thinning of bones and cartilage and joint discs. The changes in the musculoskeletal system usually associated with old age are brought on prematurely by lack of activity. It is a fundamental physiological truth that the health and nutrition of tissues like bone, cartilage and muscle are dependent on the stresses placed upon them. The body is not unlike a fine piece of complicated machinery which will slowly deteriorate if not in constant use.

Regular exercise and physical training leads to important and easily measurable changes in the cardio-respiratory and musuloskeletal systems. Such beneficial changes can take place at all but an advanced age, no matter how inactive you have been in the past.

With exercise, heart muscle strengthens and becomes more efficient and its blood supply improves. Stroke output (blood pumped per beat) and minute output (blood pumped per minute) increase substantially so that the heart's reserve capacity is greatly enhanced. The fit, well-trained heart will carry out work at a lower pulse rate and with less effort than the unfit heart. Hence the greater exercise capacity and endurance of the fit person. The fit heart is also more stable and less likely to develop serious irregularities or sudden failure.

The efficiency of the lungs improves too, with an increased maximum breathing capacity, increasing in turn the amount of oxygen available to the tissues. Regularly exercised muscle also increases in strength and stamina, thanks to an improved blood supply and to the more efficient utilization of oxygen and of the energy-supply substances, sugar and fat.

Joints which are regularly used are more stable and mobile and are better able to withstand intense and prolonged pressure and movement. Like healthy muscle and bone, they are also more likely to recover quickly from injury and strain. Bone, cartilage and sinews are also stronger and healthier, and the interplay of movement in the muscle, sinew, bone and joint is more efficient, leading to economy in movement, better balance and co-ordination.

As a bonus, physically fit people have a higher level of the protective high-density lipoprotein (see page 87) and a lower level of the stress hormone, catecholamine. They also have less 'sticky' blood and are therefore less inclined to abnormal clotting.

There are a number of simple tests which measure the efficiency of the cardio-respiratory and musculoskeletal systems. It is a startling fact that a healthy, physically fit and regularly active man of sixty years will perform these tests at least as efficiently as an inactive man of forty. It has also been shown that after the age of twenty-five years the cardio-respiratory and musculoskeletal efficiency of an active physically fit man will deteriorate by substantially less than 10 per cent per decade, while the unfit man's capacity will reduce by twice that amount or more, not taking into account an increased risk of sedentary diseases.

Some useful hints

Before discussing specific forms of exercise and exercise programmes I would like to suggest rules which should be adopted by those wishing to become physically active and fit. Like Mario Puzo, the author of *The Godfather*, who defines a hero as a guy who is very, very careful, my definition of a hero in the context of exercise is a person who is careful about himself and about others.

This type of care and consideration requires discipline. The more diciplined you are, the greater the benefits that will come from regular physical exercise. Indeed, I believe it is difficult to achieve a genuine state of physical fitness without a modicum of self-discipline.

These 'rules' are as useful to healthy people as to those who have recovered from a heart attack and they should be used by all age groups and by women as well as men. The twenty-six-mile marathon in New York in October 1978 was won by a man in two hours and ten minutes. The best woman runner did it in two hours and thirty-two minutes – a great performance considering the tremendous musculo-skeletal advantages of the man. Housework alone is too limited in its variety of movement to maintain a woman's physical or mental fitness. The same goes for gardening; tackled in the right way it is beneficial to good muscle tone – but it is not varied enough.

In most Western countries exercise and sport are dominated by competition, particularly among the young. Competition is necessary in sport but it should not dominate a community's exercise and recreational interests. Both sexes and all ages can be physically active. In 1977 a joint Common Market/World Health Organiza-tion workshop made recommendations about a more enlightened public policy, with practical suggestions to all the European governments. These recommendations included more pedestrianized streets, more bicycle pathways, more parks and forest pathways, and better recreational facilities in schools and colleges.

1. An exercise programme should be practised regularly and permanently without excessive stop/start periods. The exercise should be built up gradually at the start of the programme. Transient aches and pains in the early stages of certain activities can be ignored.

2. Except for the young, exercise should not be excessive or too competitive. The amount of time spent exercising is as important as the intensity of the exercise. Jog/walking five miles will bring the same degree of fitness as running the same distance in half the time.

There is no merit in too much exercise, which may lead to excessive weight loss. This can happen to those who become obsessed by exercise. All active people will benefit by regular rest periods, particularly after the main meal of the day or during the weekend. No matter how active you want to be, it is a good idea to take one day off every week.

3. Any form of exercise is good as long as it is safe, enjoyable and feasible. Whatever form of exercise or recreation you adopt, try to learn the proper techniques.

It is not necessary to be an expert but you will get more enjoyment and more value out of jogging if you do it properly and the same may be said about calisthenics (pages 59–62), cycling and all ball games. A few lessons from a professional and advice from other participants will be a great help. There are many books available which are helpful and informative and which deal with every form of exercise, however obscure.

4. A variety of different exercises should be included in the programme. This is particularly important for the city-dweller who is subject to many constraints and who needs to be innovative in his planning. It is also important when weather conditions are uncertain. A wide range of choice will encourage you to exercise regularly.

As a busy inner-city dweller I practise calisthenics, I jog/walk or run, play tennis and golf, cycle and do some gardening. I walk everywhere in my hospital and never use the lift. Having such a choice of exercises means that I do not get bored by any one. There is always something available even if some exercises are barred by circumstances, weather, or minor injuries. Variety will add to enjoyment and ensure total involvement of the musculoskeletal system and therefore a greater degree of flexibility and a more complete form of physical exercise.

5. Exercise should be isotonic, that is, involving movement and the use of large muscles. Isometric or muscle-tensing exercises, such as weight-lifting or press-ups, are unsuitable for the average person and should be reserved for young people and athletes in very special categories. They are specially designed to build up muscle and stamina, but they may also cause an undesirable increase in blood pressure and heart strain. Isotonic exercises are better because they are specifically designed to improve musculoskeletal function and cardio-respiratory health and efficiency.

6. Proper equipment must be used and the surroundings of the exercise should be pleasant and safe. Rain, cold, heat and other climatic circumstances do not necessar-

ily prevent regular outdoor exercise if the form of exercise is appropriate and if proper clothing and equipment are used. For instance, I have learned to enjoy running in the rain as long as I wear old clothes and non-slip shoes.

7. You should avoid exercise for an hour or two after meals and for longer after the main meal of the day. It should also be avoided after alcohol. Stop all active exercise except the lightest calisthenics during illness and during virus infections such as influenza or colds. I would, however, recommend regular light calisthenics during illness. They will accelerate the recovery phase and a return to physical fitness.

8. All forms of extreme behaviour should be avoided. Moderation in diet and medication is best. There is no virtue in being excessive in your habits. It only leads to an obsession with your health and that can't be good either for you or for those who have to listen to you. There is no better way of putting somebody off exercise than by continually preaching about it.

9. Excessively heavy or competitive physical activity may be unsafe in older people. There is substantial evidence, however, that regular, sensible exercise, leading to a high degree of physical fitness, is entirely safe providing that you do not smoke heavily and are not grossly overweight.

To be sure that you are healthy and risk free it is important to see your doctor before you start becoming active. He will check your heart, lungs and musculoskeletal system as part of his examination, and ensure that you have no obvious coronary risk factors. He may also do a few tests, including an ECG before and after exercise.

If you have been cleared by your doctor you need not be under regular medical supervision, but an occasional medical check-up, say every two to four years, is desirable for the average person. An exception here is the person who has had a previous heart attack. While he should also aim to be thoroughly fit and active, his exercise programme is best carried out under special medical supervision, particularly during the early stages of recovery.

5 OUTDOOR EXERCISE

The amount of exercise you need varies according to age and fitness. Obviously, other considerations, such as alternative forms of exercise, your habits and medical history, and your motivation must be taken into account.

If you have had a coronary heart attack, you can still be fit; fitness is a good thing for you and quite safe so long as the build-up is slow and the amount of exercise is matched to the amount of heart damage. A person with fairly extensive scarring of the heart muscle must be careful about exercising and the same goes for those who are limited by angina of effort. If, however, there is plenty of healthy heart muscle with limited scarring and, if appropriate stress tests show no adverse effects, it is perfectly feasible to exercise, at least under medical supervision.

After a heart attack you should always be more careful about becoming fit but, bearing in mind that fitness is the product of intensity over time, there is no reason why you may not be as fit as the person free from heart disease, even though it might take longer and you have to be more prudent in achieving this aim.

People who smoke cigarettes or who drink more than the average amount of alcohol, both high risks, should be prudent about their degree of activity. In fact this problem does not often arise because heavy smokers and drinkers are seldom motivated to pursue a programme of physical exercise and, if they do exercise regularly, they frequently modify their habits.

Walking, jogging and running

There is no clear cut-off point between walking, jogging and running. They can be done separately or combined in various ways and they are the basis of a good exercise programme. They are suitable for both sexes and all ages and can be done alone or with others. Except in a few built-up areas, time or place is no bar, although the urban dweller may need to drive from home to a suitable place to jog or run.

Jog/walk/running should be done regularly, irrespective of other activities. I try to jog regularly two or three times weekly. If I do it less frequently it takes greater resolution to get going.

Some of the practical problems of inner-city running, and how they can be solved, are illustrated by my own experiences. I jog or run two to four miles in twenty to forty minutes two or three times a week. I usually go out in the early morning, before breakfast, or late in the evening. The streets are less crowded then, giving me more room and a greater choice of location and making me less conspicuous. I avoid running after meals.

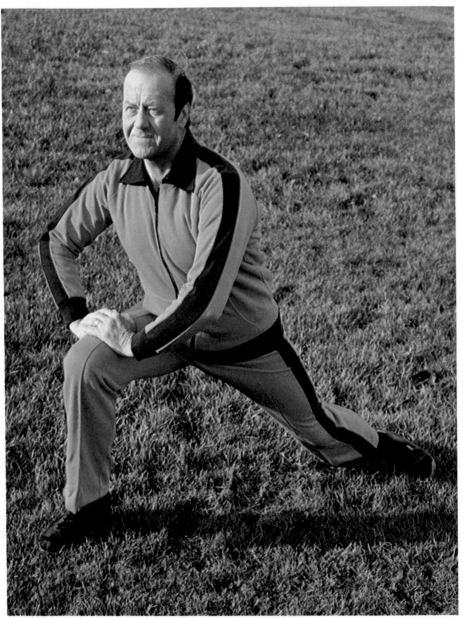

Warming up

Do some gentle stretching exercises to warm up before jogging or running. Some people like to do a few afterwards as well.

ABOVE: Bend one knee, the other leg stretched behind. Place hands together on your knee and lean forward. This exercise stretches the muscles of the inner thigh. Repeat eight to ten times on each leg.

RIGHT: Stand on one leg, raise the other knee to your chest. Repeat eight to ten times on each leg. This stretches the hamstrings in the thigh.

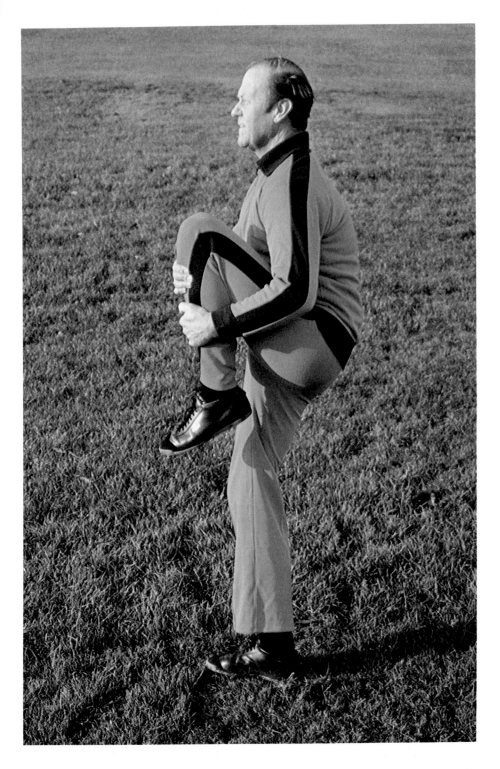

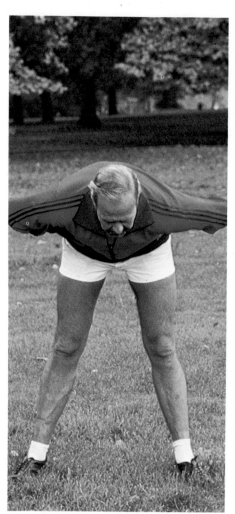
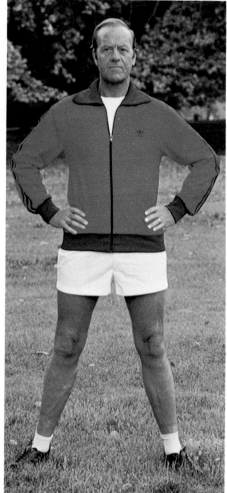

Trunk circling

To loosen up the whole torso. Lean forwards to waist level, then up straight. Bend back to the left as far as you can comfortably go, then over to the right before stretching forwards again. Repeat as often as you wish.

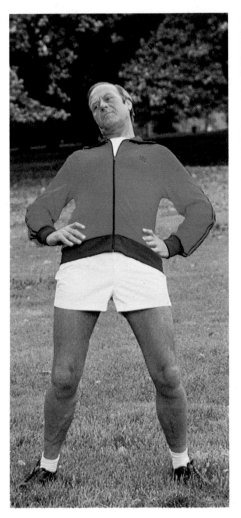 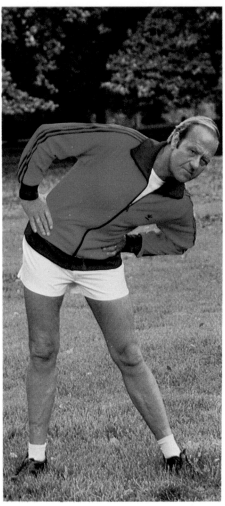

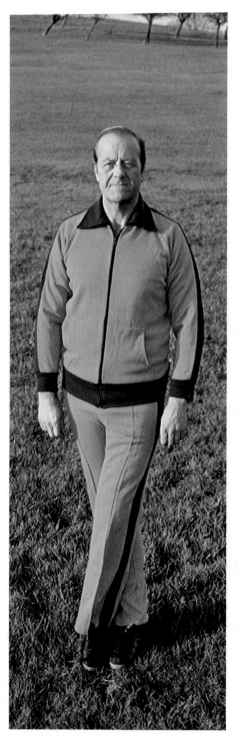

Cross-leg toe touch

Stand upright and place one foot over the other. Both legs are straight. Lean forwards as far as you can reach. This stretches the thigh muscles.

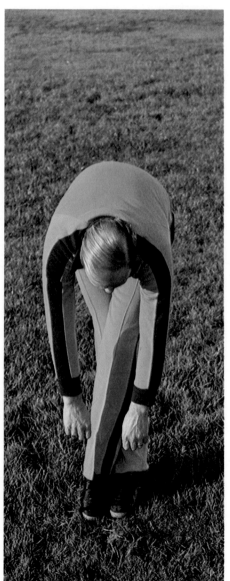

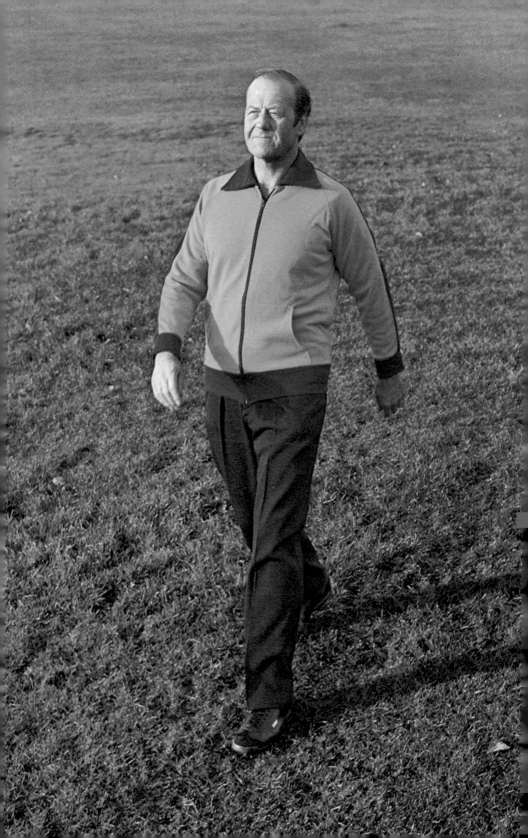

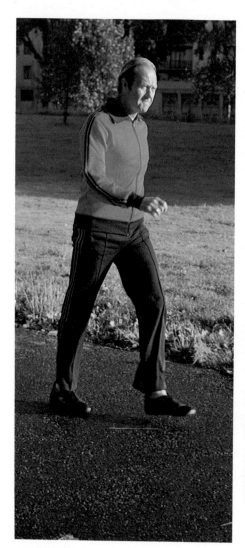
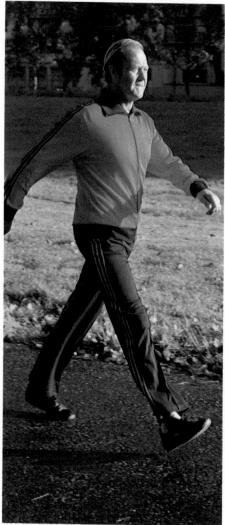

Walking

ABOVE: Always remember to 'walk tall', swinging your arms forwards and make sure you use your whole foot — heel and toe.

Taking your pulse

RIGHT: Place your fingers on the front and outer side of your wrist (don't use your thumb). Your pulse rate will go up after exercise. Always avoid over-exertion and never let your pulse go above 190 per minute minus your age.

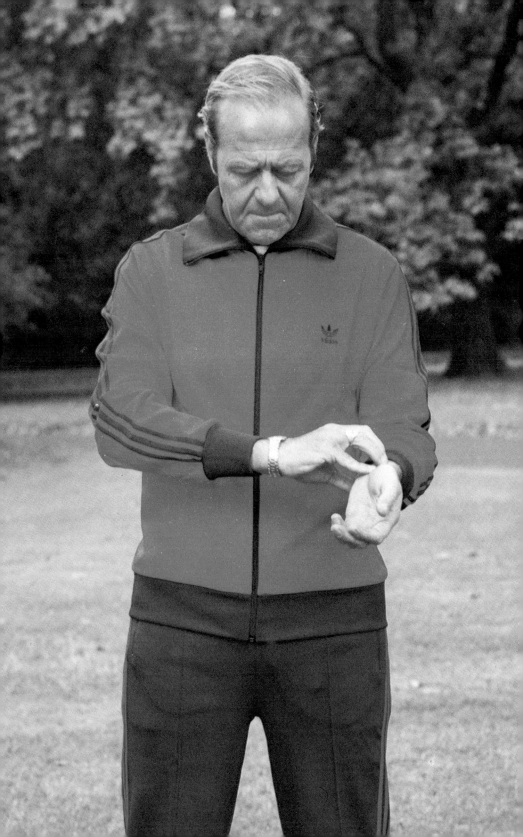

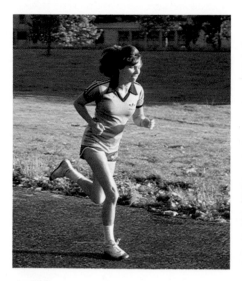
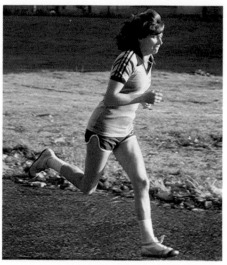

Running Run heel-toe and let your arms swing as above. Start by running for a few moments, increasing to ten or twenty minutes.

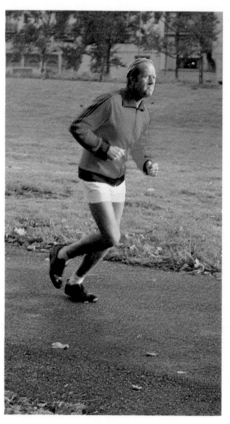
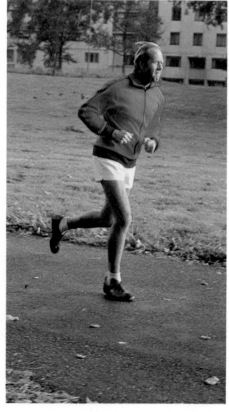

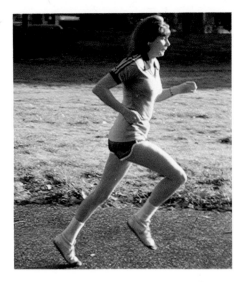 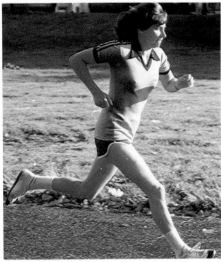

Jogging BELOW: Slower and more relaxed than running. You can also alternate it with walking.

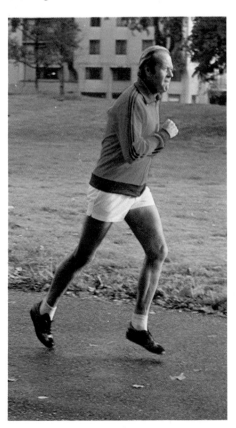 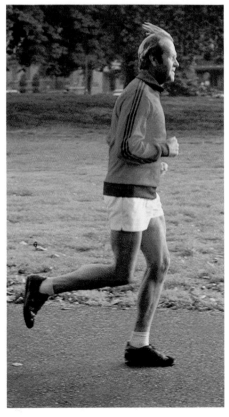

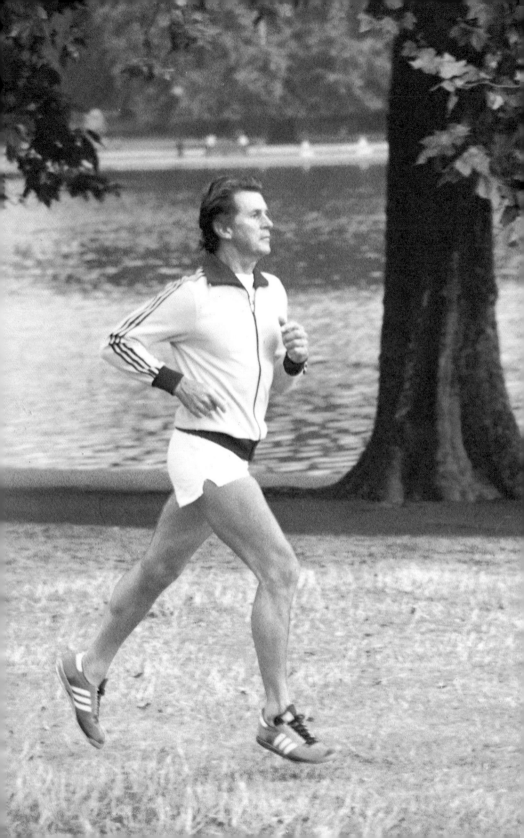

I only go to places which are well-lit at night to avoid injury on rough surfaces and encounters with undesirable citizens. For interest and variety I run in most parts of the south-eastern area of the city. By now I know not only every part of Georgian Dublin, but most of the byways and nooks and crannies of the adjacent suburbs. Apart from the joys of jog/walking and running, there is great pleasure to be gained from intimate contact with a city like Dublin and that pleasure is enhanced by the tranquil atmosphere and quiet streets at night-time and in the early morning. Wherever you live there is no better way of getting to know it than to walk or run along the streets or tracks.

I do my jogging in such a way that I am sweating fairly profusely and notice that my muscles are tired by the time I arrive home. When in good form I can jog or run continuously but I slow down to a walk when I feel any discomfort from breathlessness, chest heaviness, stitch or leg fatigue. I find that twenty to fifty steps at a walking pace allow me to jog again. Some people find track running rather boring but for a fairly quick run of half to one mile before or after other activities it is excellent.

A good rule to establish the right intensity level of exercise for you is to be able to talk without difficulty during activity. Another general rule is to avoid a rise in heart rate above 190 minus your age. I find that I do not need to count my pulse or heart rate but, without counting, I become conscious of a heavy heart action if the rate goes much above this limit.

For the first few hundred yards I walk as much as I jog, so that I start each session gradually. After returning home I find that the stretching and joint movements of calisthenics for four or five minutes relieve the general stiffness which may follow a jog/walking session.

If I have been off exercise for an unusually long period of time, I start off gradually again and ignore the pains or aches of unfamiliar exertion.

I wear ordinary, casual clothes — generally a t-shirt with an old shirt and pair of slacks. I may carry a sweater in cold weather. Thick socks and comfortable running shoes are essential and I have found a pair of soft-soled walking shoes to be excellent. After long association they fit my feet like a glove.

It is important to choose the right shoes and socks. The careful, disciplined runner will not take chances. Shoes should not be thin-soled, at least for street running, and they should have good arch support. Clothes should be comfortable, loose and reasonably light. Non-permeable or rainproof jackets, parkas or anoraks should be avoided. This is because they prevent sweat from evaporating; your clothes become drenched and there may be an undesirable rise in body temperature leading to heat stroke if your running session is prolonged.

Whether expensive running shoes are better than the cheaper variety is difficult to say. Personally, I am interested only in comfort. Practical experience of running, supplemented by reading appropriate books and seeking advice of experts will help you to satisfy your own needs as regards shoes and equipment.

It is a simple but important matter to learn the proper techniques of walking, jogging or running from the many experts and books available. If you learn to run well it will be safer and will do you more good; you may like to keep a record of your

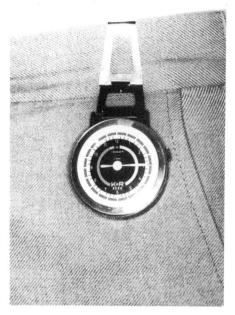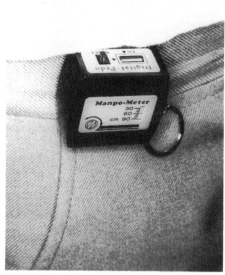

Pedometers like these show the distance covered.

activities. By using a pedometer you can estimate the distance you have jogged although, with experience, you can use your own judgement to tell you how far you have run. Pedometers are widely available and reasonably inexpensive.

Cycling

Cycling is a marvellous activity, whether you do it as a means of transport or just for fun. Not everybody will want to cycle but, for those who do, I can heartily recommend it.

Cyclists have a great advantage in that they can keep in close contact with their surroundings while reaping the benefits of fitness and of a useful and inexpensive mobility. Cycling can be enjoyed in clubs and family groups, and be the basis of vacations and weekend activity.

In recent years cycling has been enhanced by improvements in bicycles, equipment and clothing. My fairly new five-speed Raleigh racer, which is one of my proudest possessions, is so much lighter and more efficient than the 'old crock' I used to ride around Ireland during the Second World War. With its gears and light construction it is seldom necessary to get off for wind or hill, and a steady rhythm can be maintained at all times.

As far as musculoskeletal and cardio-respiratory fitness is concerned, cycling is good but the muscles in use, although large, are fairly limited. Ideally, cycling

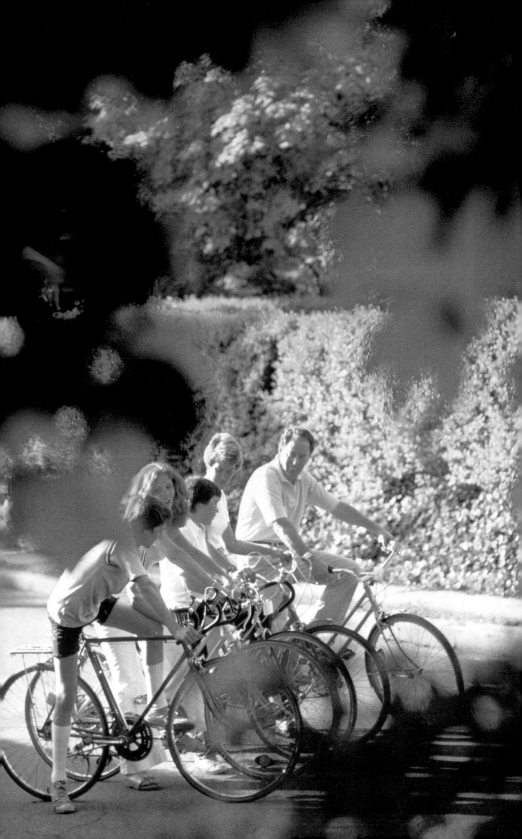

should be combined with other exercises, such as jog/walking, running and calisthenics.

If you are a keen cyclist, or intend to include cycling in your exercise programme, it is worth reading a good book about all its aspects. It is important to wear proper clothing and the benefits of cycling will be increased if you keep up a steady rhythm all the time, using your gears if necessary.

There are, of course, a number of difficulties and frustrations about cycling, particularly in the urban environment. Traffic noise and pollution are most disagreeable, particularly if the city you live in is slack about controlling them. Heavy traffic is also dangerous to cyclists no matter how considerate drivers may be and the rough surfaces of many of the roads close to footpaths add to the danger and discomfort, and are damaging to the bicycle. I don't consider cycling in towns suitable for older people. Co-ordination and quick reflexes are essential to avoid the hazards of the city and it is inevitable that senior citizens will be more vulnerable under these circumstances. Remember to keep your bicycle locked whenever it is stationary and watch out for stray dogs who may run across your path. Wear light-coloured clothes at night so motorists can easily see you.

The problems of urban traffic limit me to cycling only at night or during weekends and holidays. I am naturally conscious of the dangers in the city, even with light traffic, but I am also aware that most injuries and deaths among cyclists are caused by their own mistakes. It has been estimated in one large United States survey that more than 75 per cent of deaths among cyclists could be attributed to their breaking the rule of the road and particularly to their ignoring traffic signals. Only a minority of accidents could be attributed to motorists and others.

To avoid damage to your bike and to yourself, whether in town or country, it is essential to stick strictly to the rule of the road.

6 INDOOR EXERCISE

Calisthenics

I strongly recommend that a system of calisthenics or yoga be incorporated in every exercise programme. Calisthenics have been defined as 'gymnastic exercises designed to achieve bodily health and grace of movement'. A satisfactory system can be organized by referring to the numerous books on the subject. The object of the exercises is to carry out large joint and muscle movements such as those illustrated here. These are excellent in maintaining joint stability and mobility, and for improving muscle strength and co-ordination.

The exercises are done indoors, either without equipment or using the facilities of a gymnasium, if available. They may be practised when weather conditions prevent other forms of exercise. I find calisthenics to be a great standby when some minor injury or strain prevents me from jog/walking, cycling or playing tennis. They can be done to music. For me an average session will last out a long-playing record.

The exercises are specially designed to strengthen certain muscles and joints, and can play an important role in preventing spinal disc trouble and other sedentary, musculoskeletal problems. Combined with good posture and the right technique of lifting and bending, calisthenics, in my experience, have virtually eliminated the risk of low back pain and spinal disc trouble, even in people with chronic trouble in the past. They will also help to improve posture, movement, and the figure in various ways, such as restoring or preserving the normal spinal curve and the tone of the abdominal muscles.

Calisthenics can be practised frequently and for brief periods almost anywhere, in the office, bathroom, car, plane or even bed. They can be done regularly by the busy traveller in a hotel room or lodgings. I often practise one of the illustrated exercises when I have a spare moment or during the brief intervals which occur when playing tennis and golf. Calisthenics can be surprisingly enjoyable when you have developed a standard routine of exercise and when you do them regularly. Try to develop a sequence of exercises so that you can go through the full range of desirable movements according to a set plan.

Although calisthenics can be carried out as a group exercise, I personally enjoy them best on my own, particularly accompanied by music. I generally do the exercises in light underwear without shoes but, if in a gymnasium, wear tennis clothes and shoes. I do these exercises quite vigorously so that after about twenty minutes I am perspiring lightly, but I do not push myself to capacity and quite often have rest intervals between movements.

Skipping is another valuable form of indoor exercise and has many of the virtues of

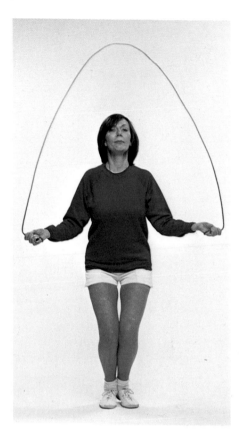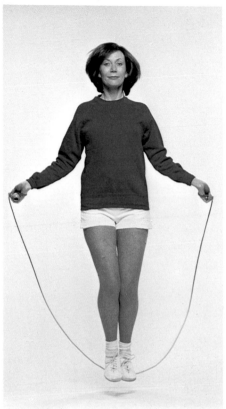

Skip rope

When skipping you move all the time – provided you don't fall over the rope! Skipping is very good for the cardio-vascular system, the pulse rate increases and more oxygen is carried through your system. Skip fifty to a hundred times. You should be panting a little at the end. Warning: skipping is strenuous so start slowly, particularly if you are middle-aged.

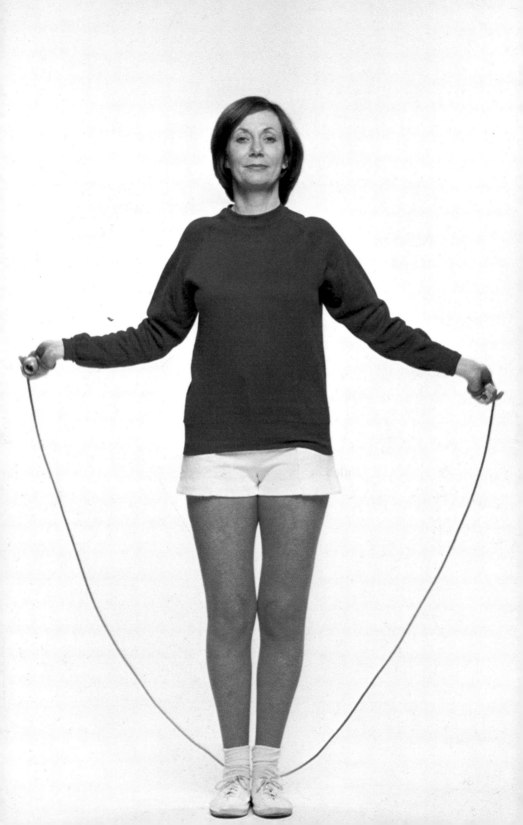

jogging and walking. It is most important that you start calisthenics and skipping exercises gradually and that you take several weeks before attaining your maximum capability.

I do the exercises at any time of the day or night, but avoid doing them after meals or after alcohol. There is a most marvellous feeling of mobility and stretching associated with these exercises which is hard for the uninitiated to appreciate. My enthusiasm for calisthenics is provoked by all these points and by the fact that I know people who keep superbly fit and youthful with regular practice and without any other form of planned exercise.

A personal exercise programme

All forms of exercise are good and many different forms of exercise are complementary. The type of exercise you practise and enjoy must depend on your own inclinations, age and possible disabilities, and on your physical and social circumstances. The city dweller has many choices of activity – I believe more than one often thinks – and the country dweller should also be well provided. In my own city area we have tennis, squash, golf, swimming, dancing, volleyball, basketball, horse riding, not to mention running, calisthenics and cycling. Skating and skiing are available in many places and it is usually easy to drive a mile or so to a local park or suburb, and also to get out to the hills and forests for climbing and walking.

My own exercise programme may be worth recounting. I rowed for three years at university and then did precious little until the age of forty, except to play golf irregularly. I took up squash at forty, became very enthusiastic and reasonably competent and played three to four times weekly. I gave up squash at fifty because I was concerned that the intense activity and the competitive nature of the game might be harmful. While I do not have access to any evidence to prove my point, I believe that excessive exercise in the fifties and sixties may be dangerous. Anyhow, I was unwilling to act as a guinea pig!

I learned to swim at forty-five with my six growing children, but I swim very little now despite having good facilities. I find it rather boring and I am not competent enough as a swimmer to be able to expend enough energy without becoming breathless and uncomfortable and frustrated by the water. For the water-lover, however, swimming is to be highly recommended as a regular exercise.

I continue to play golf but only occasionally because of the time required, but I took up tennis when I stopped playing squash. This was a very successful venture. I found tennis to be enjoyable, active, sociable and sophisticated, and sufficiently competitive to satisfy the remnants of the killer instinct which I possess. Tennis is not too time-consuming and, with the improved quality of courts and the increasing number of indoor courts, there are fewer climatic drawbacks to the game.

I also took up running and cycling about the time I stopped playing squash. I was slow to develop an interest in running because I found track running very boring, and I also tried to do too much initially. I believed at the time that I lacked the physical capacity to run. I gave up my efforts on several occasions but fortunately the

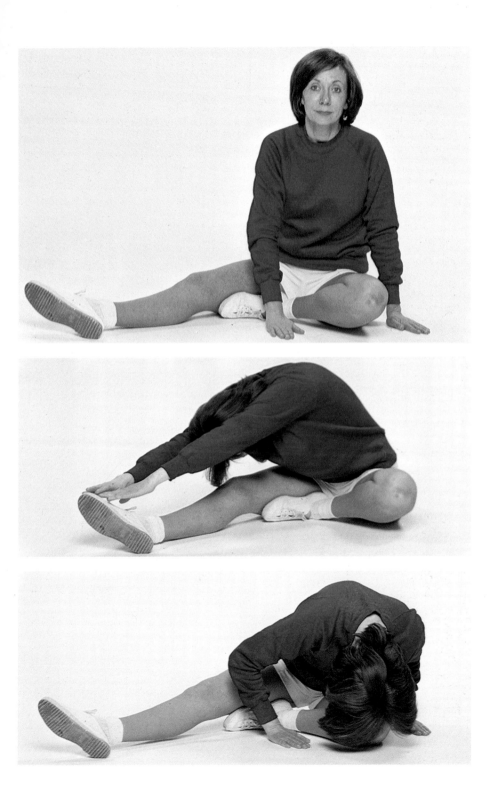

enthusiasm of some of my friends spurred me on. I have no doubt that many people fail to make the grade at running and jogging because, by starting too vigorously and impetuously, they think they are not fitted for this very natural and healthy form of exercise.

All my doubts are now resolved since I worked out a plan which suits me best. Sustained running was too strenuous but jog/walking is excellent. Track running is out, except briefly after tennis or gym, but city and country jogging are pleasant, particularly at chosen and quiet hours.

Going it alone suits me best as I find I am not distracted by other people's needs and challenges, nor by their different performances. When jog/walking or running on my own in the quiet of the morning I find a tranquil isolation and detachment which is far removed from loneliness and which is perhaps the major factor contributing to the enjoyment and euphoria of the committed runner.

This is a reminder to us that physical exercise and the pursuit of physical fitness are very personal matters. They touch on many intimate aspects of our own thoughts and emotions, including pride in body and health, and pride in one's physical and mental capacities. Exercise can hold the same contemplative significance as prayer. A dedication to exercise and physical fitness may provide an important outlet in one's life.

In my own case I can say that I have always enjoyed life, thanks as much to my leisure outlets as to my occupation as a doctor. My recent and increasing interest in exercise and physical fitness has added an important new dimension to this enjoyment, and it has also eliminated the chronic musculoskeletal problems such as recurring low back pain and cervical arthritis of which I complained up to fifteen years ago. I am completely free of these problems since I became active. In my experience others who have followed advice about physical activity and fitness have enjoyed the same benefits.

Young people often give up sport and exercise after they leave the organized and competitive environment of school and college. Older people who become committed to physical fitness will seldom stop because of the obvious physical and psychological benefits and because their motives are more personal and more compelling.

Hip flexion

PAGE 63: Bend one foot up as far as it will go, keeping your other leg straight. Stretch forwards, touching your toes if possible. After first stretch return to upright position and then bend to the other knee. Come up and repeat eight to ten times. Change to other leg. This exercise is good for the mobility of the back and hip joints.

Exercise bike

Another good exercise for the cardio-vascular system; it also increases stamina since you are moving all the time. Set the cycle for a given time or distance (two to five minutes cycling equals one to two km). If you want to work harder screw down the brakes. Make sure the saddle is at the correct height so your leg has full stretch.

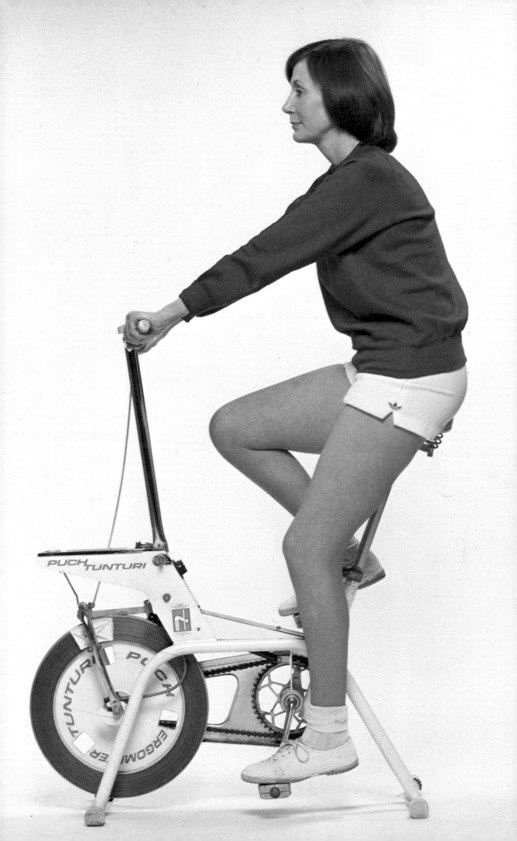

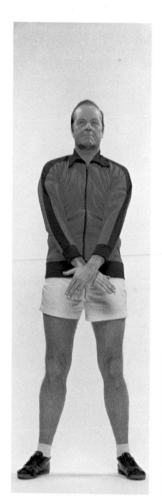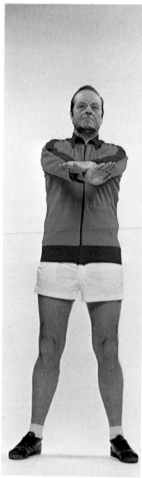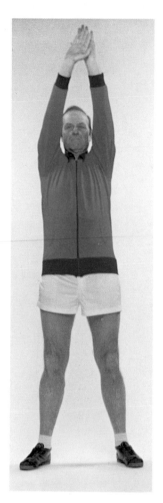

Arm circling

This exercise helps maintain the mobility and strength of the shoulder joint area and prevents stiffness and arthritis in neck and shoulders. Start by crossing your wrists in front of you, lift your arms way above your head and then out in a big, expansive movement before letting them swish down again. Remember to keep a straight back at all times. Repeat eight to ten times or more and then circle your arms in the opposite direction.

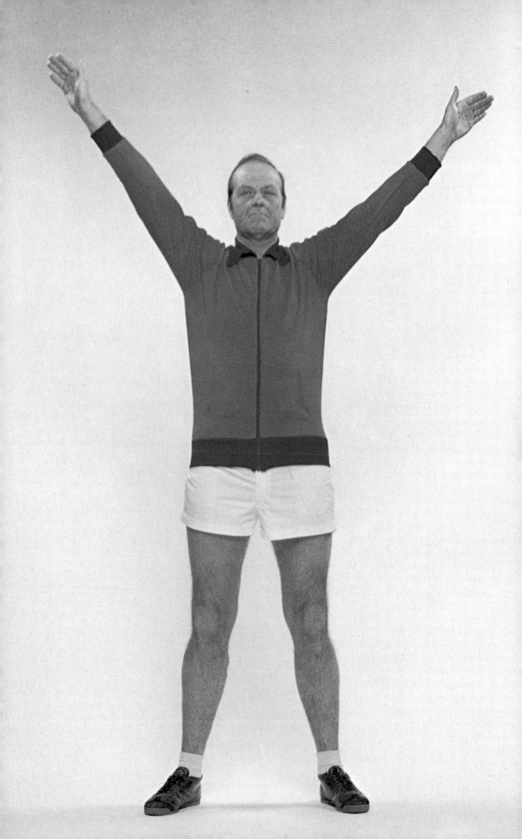

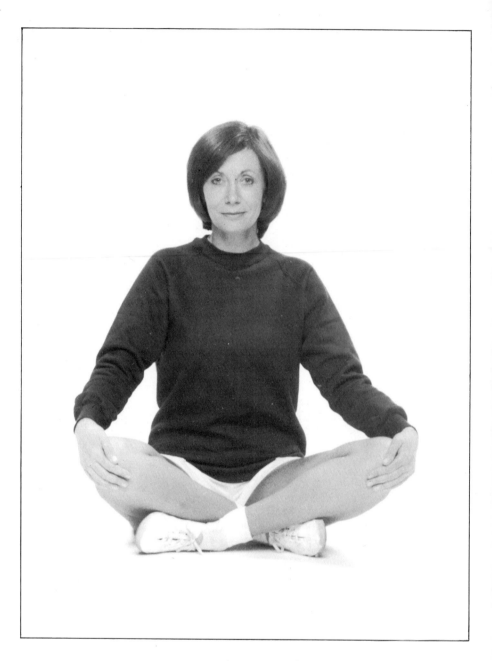

Head rolling

This stretches the neck and helps prevent neck arthritis and disc trouble. Sitting cross-legged, hands open on your knees, let your head drop back, then round to the right to drop forwards and round to the left. Keep your head rolling ten to fifteen times rhythmically and smoothly. Repeat the other way, left to right.

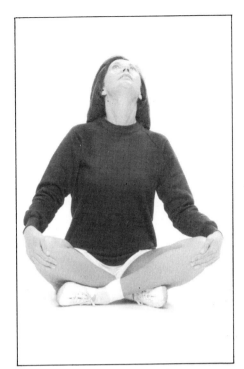

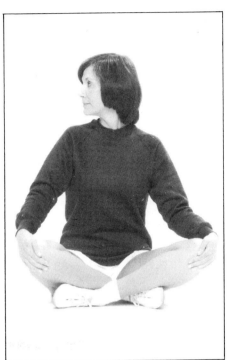

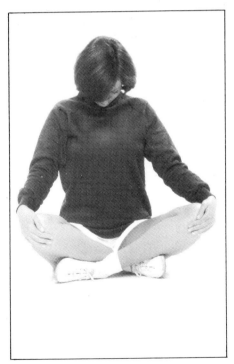

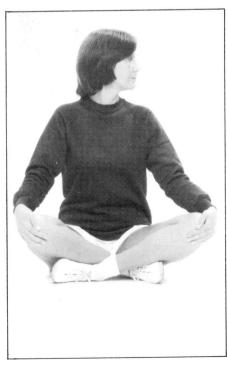

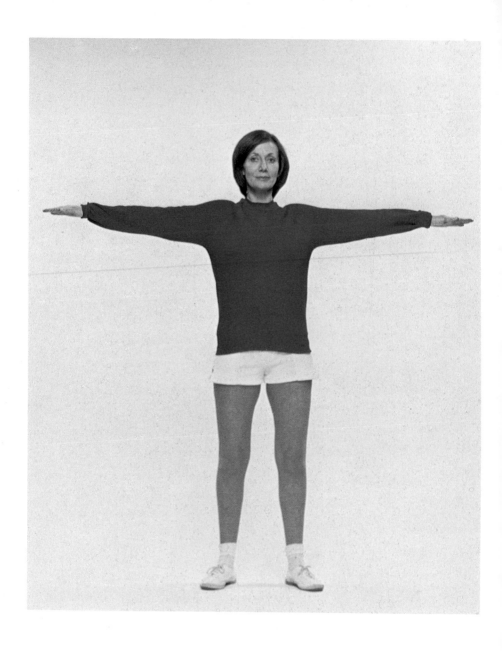

Spine bends

This is a sideways bend, starting from an upright position, which stretches the spine and dorsal muscles. Bend first to the right, come up and bend to the left. Don't bend forwards. Repeat eight to ten times.

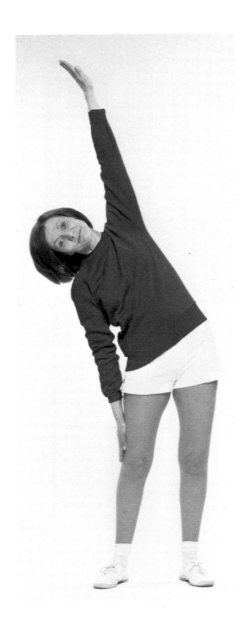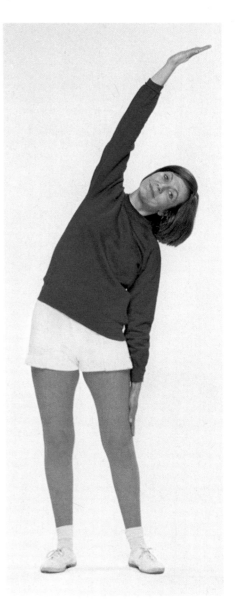

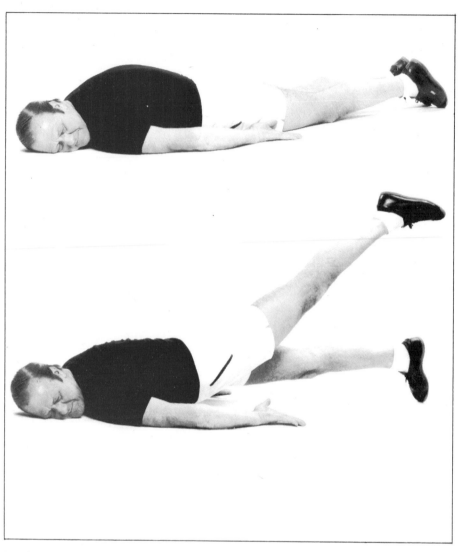

Lumbar joint – prone lying

Lie prone, keeping hips close to the floor. Raise one straight leg and keep raised for a count of three. Lower leg and repeat with other leg. Keep your palms upwards throughout. This exercise will improve your back and hip muscles and help to prevent low back trouble. Repeat eight to ten times.

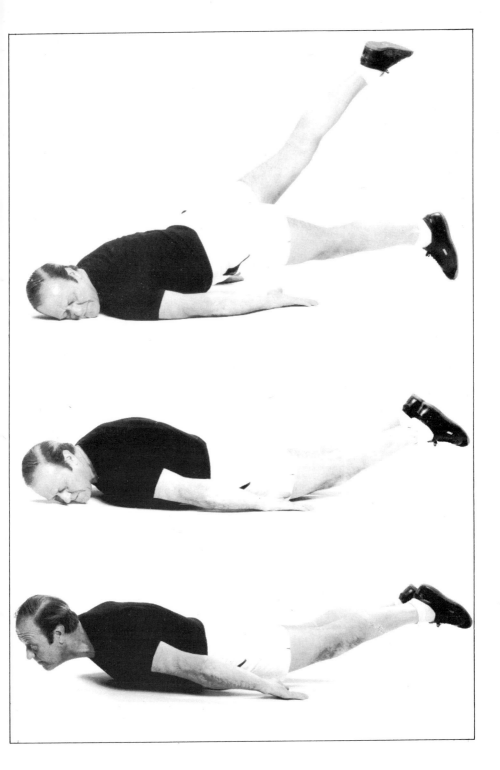

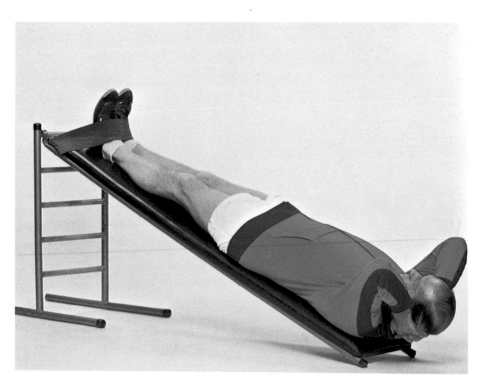

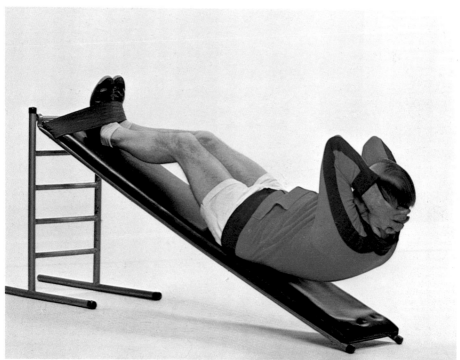

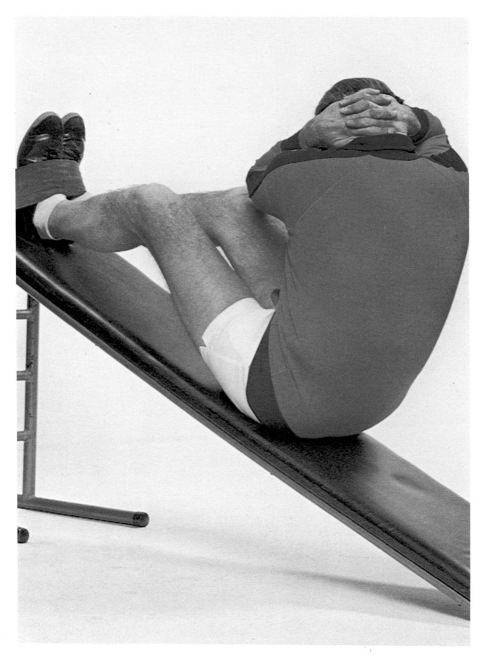

Inclined bench

An extremely strong exercise for the stomach muscles. Put the bench on the bottom rung of the ladder and gradually move up. With feet tucked behind the strap and hands behind your head raise yourself to an upright position.

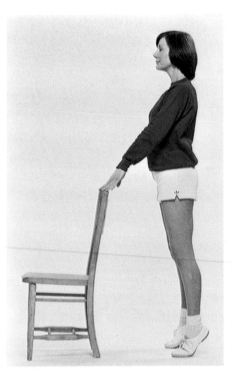 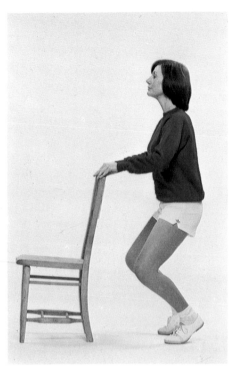

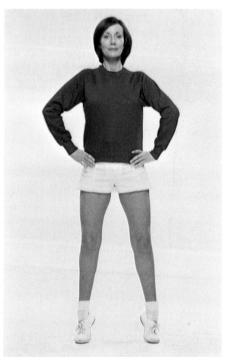 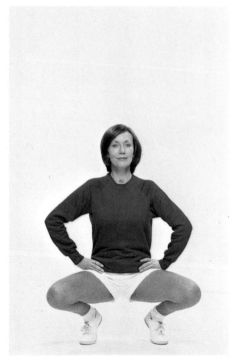

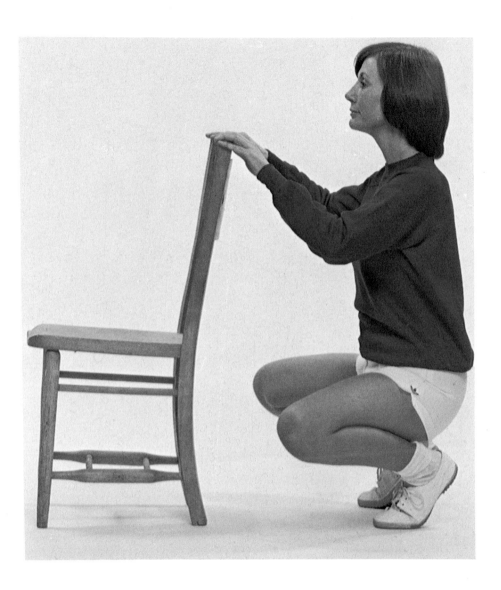

Progressive knee bends

A very strong exercise for the thigh muscles. Use a chair to start with as it helps balance. Bend down slowly, keeping your back straight, and then up smoothly on to your toes before going down again. Repeat eight to ten times. Then try without a chair.

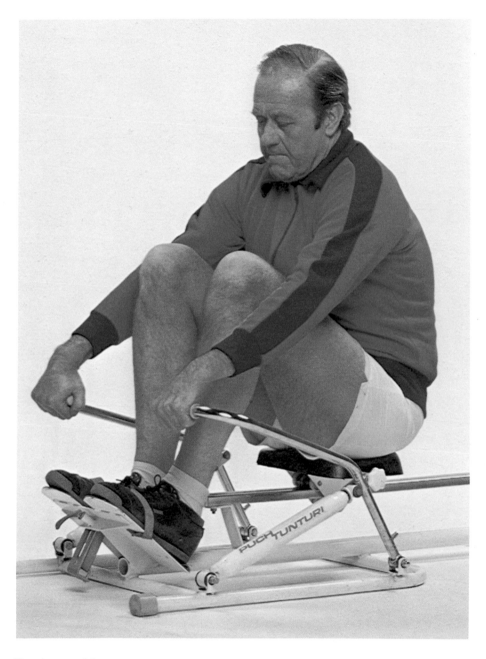

Rowing machine

This is quite strenuous and is good for the cardio-vascular system. It also increases stamina. Secure toe straps and use your legs to push and your arms and shoulders to pull. Make sure you bend your knees fully. Start gradually, increasing to about thirty strokes or a couple of minutes.

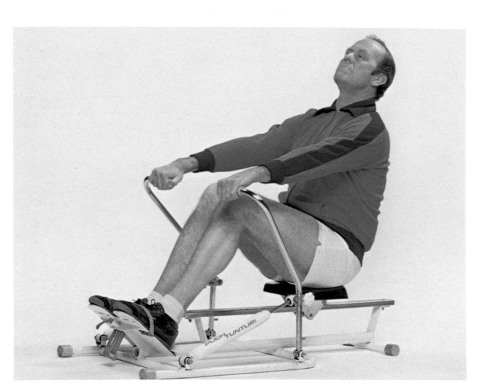

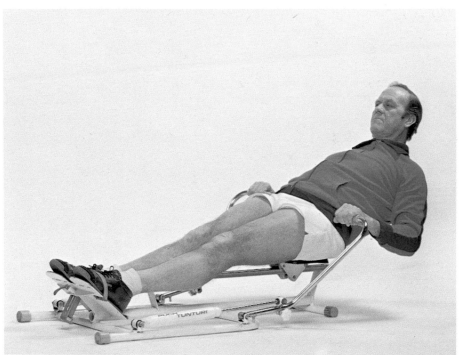

79

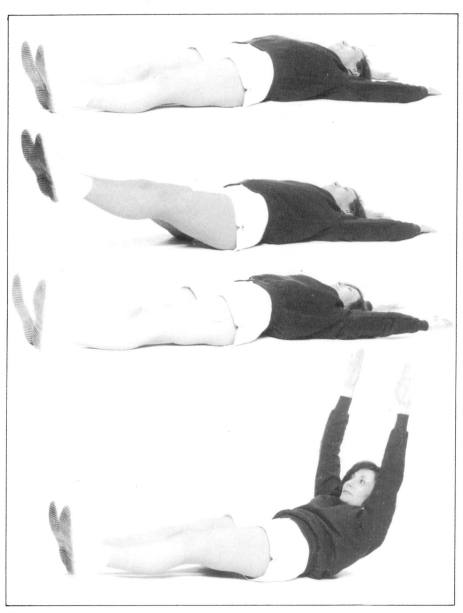

Hip joint

Strengthens the abdominal muscles and the top of the thigh muscles. Legs close
together, resting on the floor, arms stretched above your head, raise your legs slowly a
few inches off the ground. Hold for three to four seconds and lower feet. Repeat eight to
ten times.
Starting as before, swing arms up and reach forward to touch your toes, head down.
Repeat eight to ten times.
Lying down raise legs to a vertical position, bend your knees back, straighten and slowly
lower legs. Repeat eight to ten times.

80

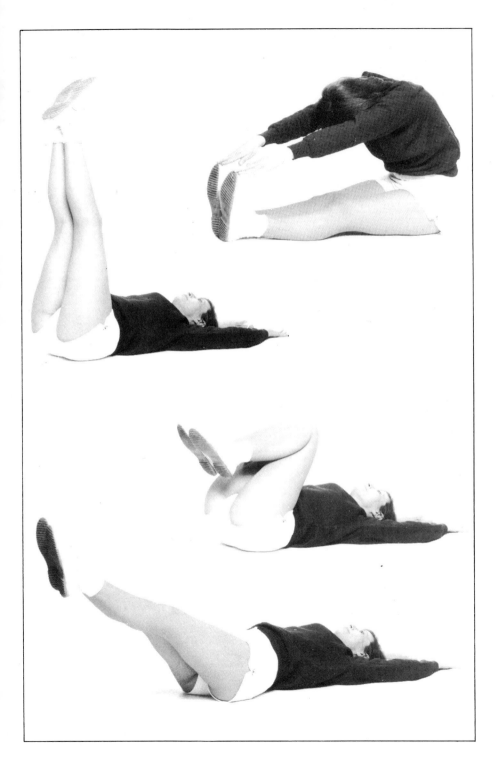

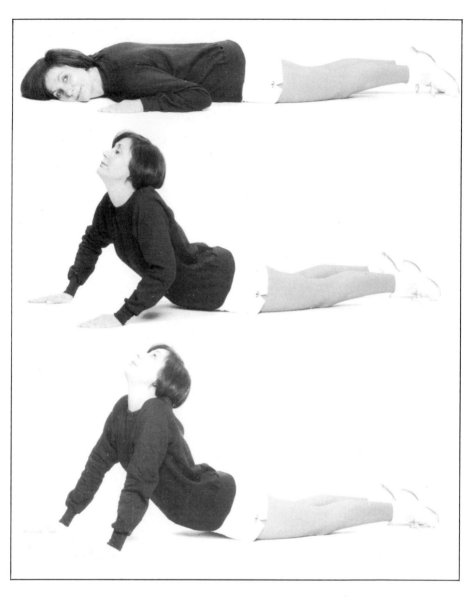

Chest raise

This is excellent for developing the lower back muscles and preventing arthritis and disc trouble. Slowly raise yourself using your lower back and buttocks. Do not push with your hands and arms; they are only to keep your balance. Keep chin and head well up. Repeat eight to ten times or more often as you get fit.

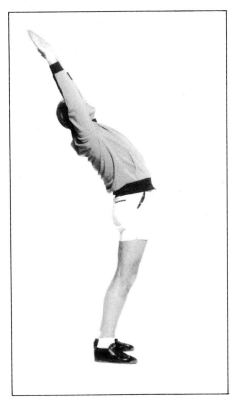

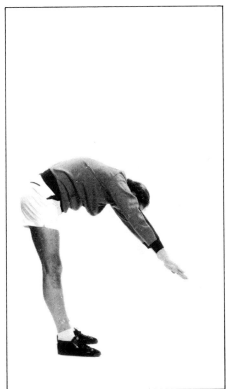

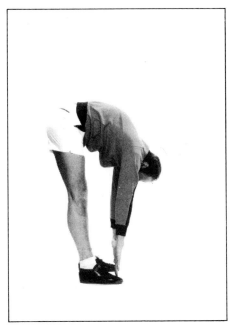

Extended toe touch

Start with feet together. Lean back slowly from your hips with outstretched arms. Count three. Flex body forward and try to touch your toes but do not strain. Return slowly to a standing position. Repeat five to ten times. This exercise is best done immediately after the knee to chest exercise (page 45). Do not attempt it if you have had recent back trouble.

7 DIET AND HEART DISEASE

Are you at risk?

Since the beginning of time malnutrition has been a major cause of disease and premature death. In the past, it implied a deficiency of energy-giving calories or an imbalance of different food constituents. Such malnutrition still exists in many developing and Third-World countries. In Western countries, however, the chief cause of malnutrition is an excessive intake of food, and particularly of certain types of food which we eat far beyond our bodily needs.

This Western form of malnutrition is a major cause of chronic disease, particularly when combined with lack of physical exercise and with an excessive intake of alcohol. We now eat too many calories, particularly in the form of sugar and high-energy foods. We eat too much animal protein and fat, and we eat too little food containing natural fibre and roughage. Most of our bad eating habits come from the increasing consumption of processed and refined food.

Common diseases associated with the Western form of malnutrition are atherosclerosis leading to coronary heart disease, stroke, and blood vessel disease in the legs and elsewhere; diabetes, obesity, gout and probably certain stomach conditions, such as gallbladder disease, colitis and pancreatitis (or inflammation of the pancreas).

No field of medicine is more open to controversy and disagreement than that of diet, mainly because it is difficult to prove anything scientifically one way or the other. Diet gives rise to many extreme views but I shall attempt to present a balanced account of the dietary aspects of heart disease — one which is based on my own experience and judgement.

It stands to reason that everybody needs to eat a well-balanced diet which contains adequate but not excessive calories, animal fat, protein, and other high-energy sucrose foods. It should also contain adequate amounts of natural fibre and other unrefined carbohydrates to give the food bulk and to make eating more palatable and satisfying. The diet should have an adequate balance of vitamins and minerals.

Cholesterol

What is it?
Cholesterol is one of the fatty substances normally present in the blood. It is essential for certain vital metabolic and energy-controlling procedures and is attached in the bloodstream to a protein particle or molecule which allows it to dissolve easily. This

eases its transport and determines its metabolic activity. An excess of cholesterol in the blood is called hypercholesterolaemia and an excess of blood fats in general is known as hyperlipidaemia. The blood fats as a whole are called lipids and they include other substances as well as cholesterol – an essential element in athero-sclerosis.

The blood fats come from two sources: either from the food we eat or from the metabolic activities of certain internal organs, such as the liver. Therefore the level of fat in the blood can be affected by the quality of diet on the one hand and by abnormal functioning of the internal organs on the other. Abnormal diet is probably the most important factor in the current high incidence of adult blood-fat distur-bances.

Determining the level of cholesterol in the blood is the simplest, least expensive and most reliable test to indicate the presence of an abnormal blood-fat level and to indicate the severity of the abnormality. It is a simple and important matter to have an occasional cholesterol check, particularly if you are at high risk for coronary disease or stroke from other causes.

Cholesterol and heart disease
There is now a vast amount of scientific evidence to link the present high incidence of atherosclerosis and its consequences with a high level of blood fats.

Three studies described here show the type of work that has established this connection:

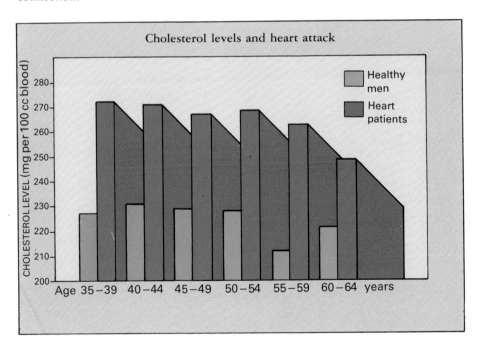

Comparison of blood cholesterol levels between 263 healthy men and 445 men who had a heart attack shows that blood cholesterol levels in these patients were significantly higher than for the healthy men.

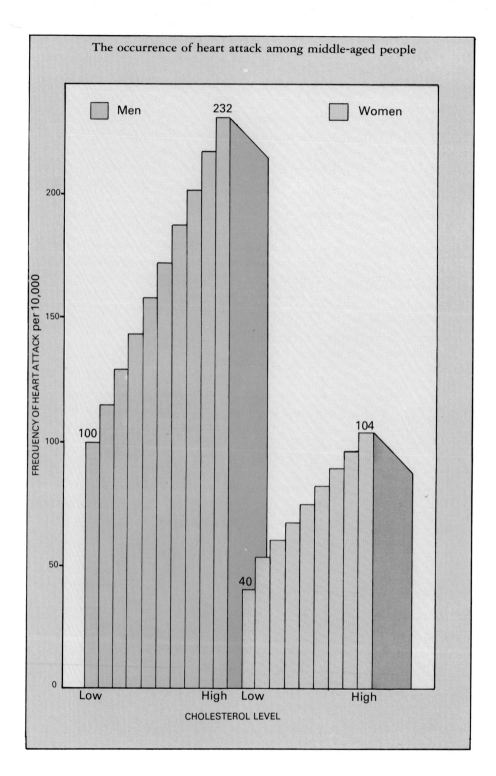

The occurrence of heart attack among middle-aged people

Men   232   Women

FREQUENCY OF HEART ATTACK per 10,000

200 —

150 —

100   104

50 —

100

40

0

Low   High   Low   High

CHOLESTEROL LEVEL

86

At my own hospital we compared the cholesterol levels of 445 men who had suffered a heart attack with the levels of 263 healthy men. This investigation showed that, for all age groups from thirty-five to sixty-five years, the patients had a cholesterol level which was substantially higher than the healthy control subjects (page 85).

At Framingham, Massachusetts in the United States, more than 5000 healthy adults had cholesterol checks more than twenty years ago as part of an important research study of coronary disease. These people have been followed up since and they are examined every two years as part of a routine check-up. The Framingham researchers have shown that those among the 5000 who subsequently developed heart attacks or stroke had substantially higher initial cholesterol levels (page 86).

In Minneapolis, Dr Ancel Keys and his colleagues carried out a similar study in seven different countries. They showed that the frequency of coronary disease was related to the average level of cholesterol in the countries and to the amount of animal-fat foods eaten by their populations.

It is interesting that atherosclerosis in animals cannot be induced without cholesterol feeding and that a regression of the disease can occur when the cholesterol-rich food is withdrawn. Also, people with a rare and severe form of hereditary cholesterol excess nearly always develop severe atherosclerosis and may suffer a heart attack as early as childhood or the early teens.

Tests for high cholesterol

The taking of a blood sample or a cholesterol estimation is a simple procedure and does not require special arrangements such as fasting beforehand. If your cholesterol is at a satisfactory level you need not have further tests. Unfortunately, not all laboratories have carefully controlled and standardized methods, but this situation is improving gradually.

If your cholesterol is found to be high, it is advisable to have further tests to determine levels of the other blood fats present and the nature of the cholesterol lipoprotein. If a substantial proportion of the cholesterol is carried in the high-density lipoproteins, the high levels may be of little consequence as there is now evidence that cholesterol carried in the high-density lipoproteins is harmless or protective compared to that attached to the low-density lipoproteins.

Examination of the other blood fats in high cholesterol states will also help determine the nature of the blood-fat abnormality and this is an essential step before proper treatment can be arranged. There are at least five different types of blood-fat disturbances, but for practical purposes these can be reduced to two: Type-2 and Type-4.

The causes of blood-fat abnormalities

A small percentage of blood-fat disturbances is hereditary in origin. These tend to be severe and difficult to treat. There is also a small number of blood-fat disturbances associated with certain medical diseases and particularly with diseases of the kidneys, liver, pancreas and thyroid gland. Treatment in these cases will depend on treating the underlying medical cause.

It may be a relief to you to know that most blood-fat and cholesterol problems are preventable and are the result of a particular life-style clearly related to bad diet, obesity and lack of exercise – or a combination of these.

It is widely reported that an excessive intake of animal fats and cholesterol-rich foods (such as dairy foods), particularly when combined with an excessive intake of calories and of high-energy foods such as sugar and meat, will lead to gradual and significant abnormalities of cholesterol and blood fats. Because these high-energy foods are the most expensive affluent populations eat more of them. This may be one reason why Western countries have a higher occurrence of atherosclerotic diseases.

There is also evidence that excessive and prolonged mental stress may contribute to increased levels and abnormal patterns of blood fats.

Some people are more susceptible to blood-fat disturbances than others. Nevertheless, the more unsatisfactory the life-style, the higher the frequency of abnormal blood fats in the community and the higher the frequency of the atherosclerotic diseases. In other words too much 'good' living can be a short-cut to a heart attack.

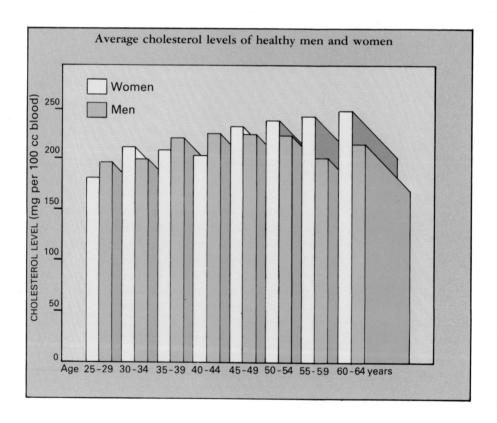

What is the difference between an abnormal and normal blood cholesterol level? It is hard to say. What is normal or average in North America is very high for a Third-World or developing country. In general, the lower the cholesterol carried in low-density lipoproteins the better. Your doctor will help you here. At relatively normal levels you should have no problem as long as you stick to a healthy diet.

Of course a coronary attack or stroke may occur in a person with low cholesterol, but it is less common and is merely a confirmation of the fact that other risk factors, such as cigarette smoking and high blood pressure, may be at fault.

Your diet

Most people with blood-fat disturbances will benefit from a change in diet. The strictness of the diet must be determined by the doctor and nutritionist for each individual. Generally you can be more easy-going if you are visiting friends and eating out as long as your usual home or family diet is followed in a satisfactory way. Half-hearted attempts to diet should be avoided – you are wasting your time and that of your advisers. Diet may have to be strict at first but, later on, when your blood fats become normal, your weight is controlled and you are exercising adequately, you can be a little less strict with yourself.

What should you eat?

If you are in any doubt about what food to eat your national heart foundation or health agency can give you information about low-fat and low-cholesterol foods, and about calorie control. There are many books available which list the important high-cholesterol, high-saturated and polyunsaturated-fat and high-calorie foods. Many of these contain a large and excellent variety of recipes specially designed for people with high cholesterol levels.

Cut down substantially on your intake of cholesterol-rich and animal-fat foods. This includes eggs, all the dairy foods and red meat such as steak and pork. It also includes rich processed foods such as paté, canned meats and savories. Try to eat more high-fibre foods such as vegetables, fruit, bran, unrefined cereals and wholemeal bread.

If, for reasons of taste and palatability, you need a substitute for butter and other fats eat the polyunsaturated fats, which are of marine or vegetable origin, as distinct from the saturated fats which are hard and mostly of animal origin. The polyunsaturated fats are soft at room temperature and do not cause the blood cholesterol to rise. In fact there is substantial evidence that they cause a fall in cholesterol levels.

Limit your intake of sugar and alcohol, particularly if you are overweight and if you have a Type-4 blood-fat disturbance. Reduce your weight to normal levels if it is excessive and increase your exercise substantially so that you become as physically fit and as trim as possible. Have occasional blood-lipid checks. Your doctor and nutritionist will guide you. Avoid stress. Some people have successfully overcome stress through yoga, transcendental meditation and other special techniques such as acupuncture.

In my experience, a prudent diet, normal weight, and physical fitness will, in the great majority of people, lead to normal blood-fat levels. The graph (page 90) shows the response of fifty-two patients with high cholesterol whom we followed at my

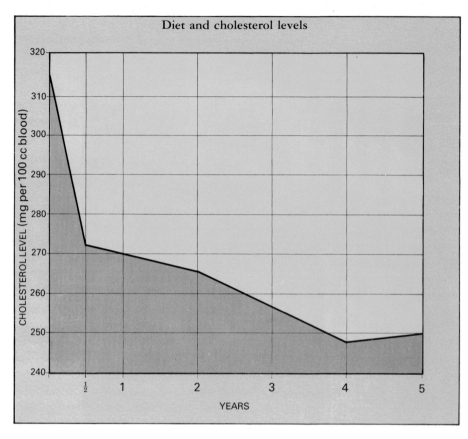

A low-cholesterol and low-fat diet reduced the high cholesterol levels in fifty-two patients over a five-year period.

hospital for five years or more. They controlled their diet and made other life-style changes. Their initially high cholesterol levels dropped by more than 20 per cent over the five years. It is obvious from this experiment, and from work done elsewhere, that a beneficial change of diet can be highly effective in lowering abnormally raised cholesterol.

What else can be done?

If your blood-fat level is too high (and a possible development of atherosclerosis is likely) you would do well to cut out other risk factors. It has been shown beyond all doubt that a combination of risk factors, such as high cholesterol and high blood pressure, or high cholesterol and cigarette smoking, increases the risk of coronary attack and stroke five to ten-fold, depending on the height of the blood pressure and the quantity of cigarettes smoked. It is essential, therefore, that if you have excessive blood fats you should stop cigarette smoking and take steps — assisted by your doctor — to control high blood pressure if it is present.

A few people appear to be resistant to natural treatment. In this case drugs may be used. When properly chosen by your doctor, drugs effectively reduce cholesterol and blood-fat levels. Unfortunately, we have only limited knowledge of the metabolic effects of these drugs and of the fate of the cholesterol removed from the blood. For example, might it be deposited in the walls of the arteries? We have no evidence that drugs reduce the frequency of heart attack. In fact, most of the evidence available would suggest that they do more harm than good. These drugs also have rather uncomfortable side-effects, particularly when taken in the large amounts that may be necessary.

Does reducing cholesterol intake help?
Some researchers report that reducing cholesterol in coronary patients is beneficial; others show no such effect. On the other hand there are no reports that lowering cholesterol naturally does any harm and it seems sensible to adopt a healthy and natural diet, to exercise regularly and to keep down your weight.

If, however, you are healthy, will reducing cholesterol have a preventive effect?

Oddly enough, this cannot be fully answered because research in this area is fraught with all types of technical and economic difficulties. A number of important field studies have been made. Some of these have failed to show any benefit but others suggest that a reduction in a community's average cholesterol level is associated with a significant reduction in the incidence of coronary heart disease.

To my mind these latter results, although not medically substantiated, conform to reason. These results are also consistent with the current situation in North America, where dietary changes in the population are associated with a small but significant reduction in average cholesterol levels and with a substantial fall in mortality from coronary disease and stroke. Although it is not yet proven that high cholesterol will always harm you, at the risk of repeating myself I would suggest that you eat animal and dairy foods in moderation. This cannot do any harm and may do much good.

8 ARE YOU OVERWEIGHT?

Obesity is the term used to describe overweight due to an excess of fat in the body. Fat is normally found under the skin and internally in the chest and abdomen. It is the energy store of the body. If you are starving, it will release calories for essential metabolic processes. Fat is derived from the various foods — carbohydrate, fat and protein — which form part of our normal diet.

The distinction between normal weight and obesity may be difficult to determine but, generally speaking, doctors consider a person obese whose weight is in excess of 15 per cent above his normal weight. I know of no way whereby a person can become obese without having a calorie intake in excess of his calorie needs.

There are no strict definitions of normal weight but the tables from the Metropolitan Life Insurance Company of New York are well-known and can be used as a guide (page 93). Using these tables as a criterion, most Western communities are overweight with an average excess among adults of about 10 per cent.

Causes of obesity

Every case of obesity can be attributed to an excess intake of calories in the form of food and alcohol over expenditure in energy. A tendency to excessive consumption of calories is aggravated by the increasingly sedentary habits of modern society and by increasing social and commercial pressures to use refined and processed foods containing high-energy sugar and fat. Obesity is also aggravated by insufficient consumption of low-energy, high-fibre foods.

Also, because high-fibre foods, such as wholemeal bread and vegetables, are bulky they fill you up more than highly refined food such as white bread.

Over-eating has become a socially accepted and, indeed, almost a socially obligatory habit in our modern consumer-orientated society. The pressures exerted by commercial interests to make us over-eat and to eat high-energy processed foods affect children at least as much as adults and have a disastrous effect on their long-term eating habits.

Over-feeding may be a throwback from the days before the Second World War when fat babies were approved of by doctors and by the public health authorities. Over-eating may also be a tradition in certain communities and religious groups.

Frequently, over-eating is the result of bad habits acquired during childhood and encouraged by parents. Pressures on children to over-eat may be a sign of emotional stress in the family group. The same may be seen after marriage when husband or

Weight table for men of 25 years and over (in indoor clothing)

Height ft in	(cm)	Small frame lb	kg	Medium frame lb	kg	Large frame lb	kg
5 1	(155)	112–120	(51–54)	118–129	(54–59)	126–141	(57–64)
5 2	(157)	115–123	(52–56)	121–133	(55–60)	129–144	(59–65)
5 3	(160)	118–126	(54–57)	124–136	(56–62)	132–148	(60–67)
5 4	(163)	121–129	(55–58)	127–139	(58–63)	135–152	(61–69)
5 5	(165)	124–133	(56–60)	130–143	(59–65)	138–156	(63–71)
5 6	(168)	128–137	(58–62)	134–147	(61–67)	142–161	(64–73)
5 7	(170)	132–141	(60–64)	138–152	(63–69)	147–166	(67–75)
5 8	(173)	136–145	(62–66)	142–156	(64–71)	151–170	(68–77)
5 9	(175)	140–150	(63–68)	146–160	(66–73)	155–174	(70–79)
5 10	(178)	144–154	(65–70)	150–165	(68–75)	159–179	(72–81)
5 11	(180)	148–158	(67–72)	154–170	(70–77)	164–184	(74–83)
6 0	(183)	152–162	(69–74)	158–175	(72–80)	168–189	(76–86)
6 1	(185)	156–167	(71–76)	162–180	(74–82)	173–194	(78–88)
6 2	(188)	160–171	(73–78)	167–185	(76–84)	178–199	(81–90)
6 3	(190)	164–175	(74–80)	172–190	(78–86)	182–204	(83–92)

Weight table for women aged 25 and over (in indoor clothing)

(For women aged between 18 and 25 subtract 1 lb ($\frac{1}{2}$ kg) for each year under 25)

Height ft in	(cm)	Small frame lb	kg	Medium frame lb	kg	Large frame lb	kg
4 8	(142)	92–98	(42–44)	96–107	(44–49)	104–119	(47–54)
4 9	(145)	94–101	(43–46)	98–110	(45–50)	106–122	(48–55)
4 10	(147)	96–104	(44–47)	101–113	(46–51)	109–125	(49–57)
4 11	(150)	99–107	(45–48)	104–116	(47–53)	112–128	(51–58)
5 0	(152)	102–110	(46–50)	107–119	(48–54)	115–131	(52–59)
5 1	(155)	105–113	(48–51)	110–122	(50–55)	118–134	(53–60)
5 2	(157)	108–116	(49–53)	113–126	(51–57)	121–138	(55–63)
5 3	(160)	111–119	(50–54)	116–130	(53–59)	125–142	(57–64)
5 4	(163)	114–123	(52–56)	120–135	(54–61)	129–146	(58–66)
5 5	(165)	118–127	(53–58)	124–139	(56–63)	133–150	(60–68)
5 6	(168)	122–131	(55–59)	128–143	(58–65)	137–154	(62–70)
5 7	(170)	126–135	(57–61)	132–147	(60–67)	141–158	(64–72)
5 8	(173)	130–140	(59–63)	136–151	(62–69)	145–163	(66–74)
5 9	(175)	134–144	(61–65)	140–155	(63–70)	149–168	(68–76)
5 10	(178)	138–148	(63–67)	144–159	(65–72)	153–173	(69–78)

wife (or both), for emotional or other reasons, dramatically alter their eating habits.

In my view the commonest cause of over-eating is physical and mental boredom. This is particularly common among housewives who find themselves alone in the house all day with not much company or outside stimulation. Eating may be the housewife's only solace and, in extreme cases, her only means of relieving her tensions and frustrations. It is well known that depressed and anxious people are also prone to eat to excess.

A major cause of obesity, particularly among men, is too much alcohol. Alcohol is a high-energy food which can add substantially to your calorie intake. It stimulates your appetite and so may cause you to eat more. When I see a fat man I usually know that he drinks fairly heavily and that he has a caring wife who feeds him well.

Why do so many people eat too much? Or, to put in another way, if you are overweight why do you eat more than you need? Find the answer to that question and it will be much easier to lose weight and to lose it permanently. You must identify the cause of your over-eating and yet it is the exception rather than the rule for doctors and patients to get down to the basic causes. If the cause of over-eating can be identified, either by you or by your doctor, and if you really want to lose weight, it will be much easier to do so. Likewise, if a man needs to lose weight his wife should be brought into the picture from the start. It is no good his going on a diet if she insists on over-feeding him.

You should be aware that losing weight isn't all plain sailing; you may suffer as a result, particularly if you lose weight rapidly from an excessively strict diet. Depression, for instance, can be worsened if a person's only source of comfort is removed without providing a substitute. Also, very rapid weight reduction in very obese people can be physically dangerous and sometimes causes serious or even fatal biochemical changes in the blood.

Obesity has a number of disadvantages: personal, social and medical. In general, a fat person is more liable to various sedentary and musculoskeletal disorders and is therefore more likely to be off work, sick and disabled. He tends to be accident-prone and to develop more complications and recover more slowly after accidents and operations. A fat person's expectation of life is also reduced and, as the World Health Organization has pointed out, this reduction is directly related to the degree of obesity (page 95).

High blood pressure, blood-fat disturbances and diabetes are commoner in obese people. In fact, insurance statistics show that mortality from all causes is greater in obese people – and this includes the commonest causes of serious illness and premature death in our society: coronary heart disease and stroke.

What you can do to reduce weight

The one good thing about obesity is that (expect in a few rare cases) it need not be permanent. If you are fat, however, you must alter your attitude towards food if you are to improve your eating habits. This may require a fundamental change in life-style. Crash diets are futile if the cause of over-eating is not appreciated. Many

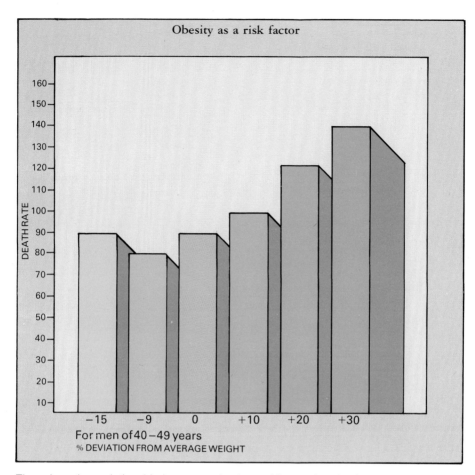

Obesity as a risk factor

DEATH RATE

For men of 40–49 years
% DEVIATION FROM AVERAGE WEIGHT

There is a clear relationship between obesity and increasing death rates. The average death rate for the population is 100.

extreme diets are advocated because they lead to a reduced calorie intake, but in my experience they are seldom successful in the long run.

It's a good idea to know the calorie values of all the common foods. This means you can substitute low-calorie high-residue foods for sugar, fat and high-energy foods. Cut down on alcohol, or preferably cut it out altogether. At least avoid the appetite-stimulating effects of alcohol by not drinking before meals. If you need further advice, enlist the assistance of a nutritionist. The accompanying calorie table is not exhaustive but will help you to choose your food wisely.

Drastic and rapid weight reduction is not necessary if you have developed the right attitude and approach to weight control. A gradual reduction is best and it is reassuring to know that, when you have achieved your desired weight, you can be more liberal in your food and alcohol intake.

OVERLEAF: Hiking can help you keep in good shape and relax at the same time.

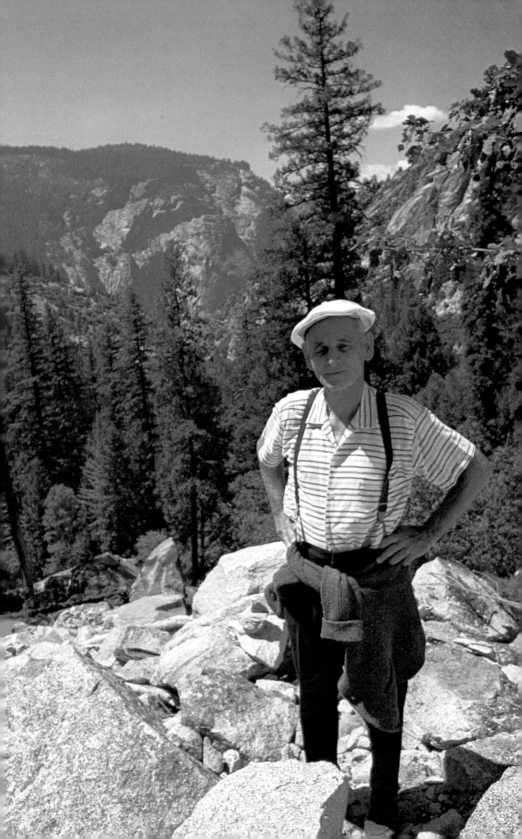

Guide to calorie values for the UK, Ireland and Australia

Dairy products

	Calories
Butter *1 oz (30 g)*	220
Cheese, Cheddar *1 oz (30 g)*	120
cream *1 oz (30 g)*	100
low fat, cottage *1 oz (30 g)*	30
thickened *1 oz (30 g)*	95
reduced *1 oz (30 g)*	80
Egg fried or scrambled *2 oz (60 g)*	135
poached or boiled *2 oz (60 g)*	93
Low-fat spread *1 oz (30 g)*	105
Margarine *1 oz (30 g)*	220
Milk, dried, skimmed *1 oz (30 g)*	95
fresh, skimmed *½ pt (300 ml)*	100
fresh, whole *½ pt (300 ml)*	190
Yogurt flavoured *1 oz (30 g)*	30
natural *1 oz (30 g)*	20
natural, non-fat *1 oz (30 g)*	15

Meat and poultry

	Calories
Bacon, grilled *4 oz (125 g)*	700
gammon rashers *4 oz (125 g)*	520
Beef corned *4 oz)125 g)*	280
roast, lean *4 oz (125 g)*	255
steak, grilled *4 oz (125 g)*	330
Chicken, av roast *4 oz (125 g)*	250
boiled *4 oz (125 g)*	220
Duck, roast *4 oz (125 g)*	350
Frankfurters *4 oz (125 g)*	290
Goose, roast *4 oz (125 g)*	370
Ham, lean, boiled *4 oz (125 g)*	250
Hamburger *1 medium*	125
Kidneys, grilled *4 oz (125 g)*	130
Lamb, chop, lean, grilled *4 oz (125 g)*	310
chop, fried *4 oz (125 g)*	340
Lamb, av roast *4 oz (125 g)*	450
lean, dry roast *4 oz (125 g)*	350
Liver, grilled *4 oz (125 g)*	180
Pork chop, lean, grilled *4 oz (125 g)*	400
Sausages, beef, thick, grilled *4 oz (125 g)*	280
pork, thick, grilled *4 oz (125 g)*	330
Sausage roll *4 oz (125 g)*	300
Tongue *4 oz (125 g)*	115
Tripe *4 oz (125 g)*	125
Turkey, av roast *4 oz (125 g)*	340
dry roast *4 oz (125 g)*	240
Veal *4 oz (125 g)*	220

Fish

	Calories
Bream *4 oz (125 g)*	160
Cod, fillets, baked *4 oz (125 g)*	95
fillets, grilled *4 oz (125 g)*	95
Flounder *4 oz (125 g)*	120
Haddock, smoked, poached *4 oz (125 g)*	128
Halibut *4 oz (125 g)*	160
Herring, fried *4 oz (125 g)*	270
grilled *4 oz (125 g)*	190
tinned, plain *4 oz (125 g)*	250
tinned, in tomato sauce *4 oz (125 g)*	220
Kipper grilled *4 oz (125 g)*	200
Lobster *4 oz (125 g)*	115
Mackerel, grilled *4 oz (125 g)*	200
Oysters *½ doz*	40
Pilchard, tinned *4 oz (125 g)*	180
Plaice, steamed *4 oz (125 g)*	100
Prawns *4 oz (125 g)*	100
Salmon, fresh *4 oz (125 g)*	160
tinned *4 oz (125 g)*	160
Sardines, tinned *4 oz (125 g)*	320
Scallops *4 oz (125 g)*	100
Shrimps, fresh *4 oz (125 g)*	110
Snapper *4 oz (125 g)*	120
Sole, steamed *4 oz (125 g)*	90
Trout *4 oz (125 g)*	160
Tuna, tinned, in oil, drained *4 oz (125 g)*	225
tinned, in brine, drained *4 oz (125 g)*	150
Whiting, boiled *4 oz (125 g)*	120

Vegetables

	Calories
Asparagus *4 oz (125 g)*	20
Aubergines *4 oz (125 g)*	30
Avocado pear, half *medium*	185
Beans, baked, tinned *4 oz (125 g)*	130
broad *4 oz (125 g)*	50
French, boiled *4 oz (125 g)*	40
runner, boiled *4 oz (125 g)*	40
Beetroot, boiled *4 oz (125 g)*	40
Broccoli, boiled *4 oz (125 g)*	30
Brussel sprouts, boiled *4 oz (125 g)*	50
Cabbage, boiled *4 oz (125 g)*	30
Capsicum *4 oz (125 g)*	45
Carrots, boiled *4 oz (125 g)*	40
Cauliflower, boiled *4 oz (125 g)*	30
Celery, raw *4 oz (125 g)*	20
Cucumber *4 oz (125 g)*	20
Leeks *4 oz (125 g)*	50
Lettuce *4 oz (125 g)*	20
Mushrooms, grilled *4 oz (125 g)*	35
Onions, boiled *4 oz (125 g)*	40
Parsley *4 oz (125 g)*	Nil
Parsnips, boiled *4 oz (125 g)*	80
Peas, fresh, boiled *4 oz (125 g)*	90
tinned, drained *4 oz (125 g)*	100
Potatoes, boiled *4 oz (125 g)*	90
chipped, fried *4 oz (125 g)*	270
crisps *4 oz (125 g)*	680
Radish *4 oz (125 g)*	20
Spinach, boiled *4 oz (125 g)*	30
Sweetcorn *4 oz (125 g)*	105
Tomatoes, fresh *4oz (125 g)*	20
Turnips, boiled *4 oz (125 g)*	35
Watercress *4 oz (125 g)*	25

	Calories
Fruit	
Apple, baked *1 large*	100
fresh *1 medium (150 g)*	85
Apricot, dried *4 oz (125 g)*	300
Banana *1 medium (150 g)*	125
Cantaloupe melon *4 oz (125 g)*	35
Cherries, fresh *4 oz (125 g)*	90
Currants, dried *4 oz (125 g)*	320
Dates, pitted *4 oz (125 g)*	350
Figs, dried *4 oz (125 g)*	320
fresh *4 oz (125 g)*	100
Grapefruit, canned *4 oz (125 g)*	90
fresh *4 oz (125 g)*	50
Grapes *4 oz (125 g)*	80
Orange, fresh *4 oz (125 g)*	60
Peach, fresh *4 oz (125 g)*	50
tinned, sweetened *4 oz (125 g)*	85
Pineapple, fresh *4 oz (125 g)*	65
Plums, fresh *4 oz (125 g)*	75
Prunes, stewed *4 oz (125 g)*	220
Raisins, dried *4 oz (125 g)*	320
Raspberries, fresh *4 oz (125 g)*	70
Strawberries, fresh *4 oz (125 g)*	45
Sultanas, dried *4 oz (125 g)*	320
Watermelon *4 oz (125 g)*	30

Puddings	
Blancmange *4 oz (125 g)*	140
Custard *4 oz (125 g)*	130
Ice Cream *4 oz (125 g)*	220
Jelly *4 oz (125 g)*	90
Rice pudding *4 oz (125 g)*	170
Sago pudding *4 oz (125 g)*	185
Semolina pudding *4 oz (125 g)*	400
Trifle *4 oz (125 g)*	180

Biscuits, breads, cakes and cereals	
Biscuits, chocolate *2 oz (60 g)*	260
crispbread *2 oz (60 g)*	215
sweet *2 oz (60 g)*	260
Bread, brown *1 oz (30 g)*	70
white *1 oz (30 g)*	70
Cake, cheese *4 oz (125 g)*	350
fruit *2 oz (60 g)*	215
sponge *2 oz (60 g)*	185
Cereals, Allbran *1 oz (30 g)*	90
cornflakes *1 oz (30 g)*	105
oatmeal *1 oz (30 g)*	115
porridge *5 oz (155 g)*	85

	Calories
Doughnuts *2 oz (60 g)*	225
Dumplings *2 oz (60 g)*	120
Flour, cornflour *1 oz (30 g)*	100
white *1 oz (30 g)*	100
wholemeal *1 oz (30 g)*	100
Macaroni, boiled *2 oz (60 g)*	65
Pastries *2 oz (60 g)*	250
Rice, boiled *2 oz (60 g)*	70
Scones *2 oz (60 g)*	210
Spaghetti, boiled *2 oz (60 g)*	65
Yorkshire pudding *2 oz (60 g)*	75

Miscellaneous	
Chocolate *1 oz (30 g)*	160
Gravy, thick *1 teaspoon*	35
Honey, jam and syrup *1 tablespoon*	75
Mayonnaise *1 tablespoon*	80
Peanuts, shelled *1 oz (30 g)*	170
Soup, clear *1 bowl (250 ml)*	35
thick *1 bowl (250 ml)*	100
Sugar *½ oz (15 g)*	55

Drinks	
1. Alcohol	
Beer *½ pt 10 fl oz (300 ml)*	120
Champagne *10 fl oz (300 ml)*	245
Cider *½ pt 10 fl oz (300 ml)*	120
Gin, whisky, brandy, rum *1 fl oz (30 ml)*	65
Liqueurs *1 fl oz (30 ml)*	110
Sherry, sweet *1 fl oz (30 ml)*	45
dry *1 fl oz (30 ml)*	35
Stout *10 fl oz (300 ml)*	120
Wine, red *10 fl oz (300 ml)*	250
white, dry *10 fl oz (300 ml)*	230

2. Non-alcoholic drinks	
Cocoa, with milk *1 cup (250 ml)*	185
Coffee, black *1 cup (250 ml)*	Negligible
milk and sugar (1 tspn) *1 cup (250 ml)*	40
Orange juice, fresh *1 glass (150 ml)*	65
Soft drinks *1 glass (150 ml)*	80
Tea, milk and sugar (1 tspn) *1 cup (250 ml)*	40
milk, no sugar *1 cup (250 ml)*	20
Tomato juice *1 glass (150 ml)*	30

98

Guide to calorie values for North America

1 cup equals 8 fluid ounces, 3 teaspoons (tsp) equal 1 tablespoon (tbs), 4 tablespoons (tbs) equal $\frac{1}{4}$ cup.

Dairy products

	Calories
Butter *1 tbs*	95
Cheese American Cheddar *1 cube*	
$\frac{1}{8}$ in sq	
or *3 tbs grated*	110
cottage *5 tbs*	100
cream *2 tbs*	100
Cream light *2 tbs*	65
heavy *2 tbs*	120
Custard boiled or baked $\frac{1}{2}$ *cup*	130
Egg *1 medium size*	75
Margarine *1 tbs*	100
Milk buttermilk (fat free) *1 cup*	85
condensed *1$\frac{1}{2}$ tbs*	100
evaporated $\frac{1}{2}$ *cup (1 cup*	
diluted)	160
whole milk, fresh *1 cup*	170
yoghurt, plain *1 cup*	120–160

Meat and poultry

	Calories
Bacon *2–3 long slices, cooked*	100
Bacon fat *1 tbs*	100
Beef corned *1 slice 4 x 1$\frac{1}{2}$ x 1 in*	100
dried *2 oz*	100
hamburger *1 patty (3 oz)*	300
round, lean *1 med slice (2 oz)*	125
sirloin, lean *1 av slice (3 oz)*	250
tongue *2 oz*	125
Chicken broiled $\frac{1}{2}$ *med broiler*	270
roast *1 slice 4 x 2$\frac{1}{2}$ x $\frac{1}{4}$ in*	100
Frankfurter *1 sausage*	125
Ham, lean *1 slice 4$\frac{1}{4}$ x 4 x $\frac{1}{2}$ in*	265
Lamb, roast *1 slice 3$\frac{1}{2}$ x 4$\frac{1}{2}$ x $^1/_8$ in*	100
Lard *1 tbs*	100
Liver *1 slice 3 x 3 x $\frac{1}{2}$ in*	100
Liverwurst *2 oz*	130
Pork chop, lean *1 med*	200
Turkey, lean *1 slice 4 x 2$\frac{1}{2}$ x $\frac{1}{4}$ in*	100
Veal, roast *1 slice 3 x 3$\frac{3}{4}$ x $\frac{1}{2}$ in*	120

Fish

Clams, *6 round*	100
Cod-steak, *1 piece 3$\frac{1}{2}$ x 2 x 1 in*	100
Halibut, *1 piece 3 x 1$^3/_8$ x 1 in*	100
Oysters, *5 med*	100
Salmon, canned $\frac{1}{2}$ *cup*	100
Sardines, drained *5 fish 3 in long*	100
Tuna fish, canned $\frac{1}{4}$ *cup drained*	100

Vegetables

Asparagus, fresh or canned *5 stalks*	
5 in long	15
Avocado, $\frac{1}{2}$ *pear*	185
Beans, dried $\frac{1}{2}$ *cup, cooked*	135
lima, fresh or canned $\frac{1}{2}$ *cup*	100
Beet greens $\frac{1}{2}$ *cup cooked*	30
Beets *2 beets 2 in diam*	50
Broccoli *3 stalks 5$\frac{1}{2}$ in long*	100
Brussel sprouts *6 – 1$\frac{1}{2}$ in in diam*	50

	Calories
Cabbage, cooked $\frac{1}{2}$ *cup*	40
raw *1 cup*	25
Carrots, 1 carrot *4 in long*	25
Cauliflower $\frac{3}{4}$ *of a head 4$\frac{1}{4}$ in in diam*	25
Celery *2 stalks*	15
Chinese cabbage *1 cup raw*	20
Cooking fats, vegetable *1 tbs*	100
Cucumber $\frac{1}{2}$ *med*	10
Endive *average serving*	10
Kale $\frac{1}{2}$ *cup, cooked*	50
Lettuce *2 lge leaves*	5
Mushrooms *10 lge*	10
Onions *3–4 medium*	100
Parsnips *1 parsnip 7 in long*	100
Peas, canned $\frac{1}{2}$ *cup*	65
fresh shelled $\frac{3}{4}$ *cup*	100
Pepper, green *1 medium*	20
Potato chips *8–10 lge*	100
Potato salad with mayonnaise $\frac{1}{2}$ *cup*	200
Potatoes, mashed $\frac{1}{2}$ *cup*	100
sweet $\frac{1}{2}$ *medium*	100
white *1 medium*	100
Radishes *5*	10
Sauerkraut $\frac{1}{2}$ *cup*	15
Spinach $\frac{1}{2}$ *cup, cooked*	20
Squash, summer $\frac{1}{2}$ *cup, cooked*	20
winter $\frac{1}{2}$ *cup cooked*	50
Tomatoes, canned $\frac{1}{2}$ *cup*	25
fresh *1 medium*	30
Turnip *1 – 1$\frac{3}{4}$ in in diam*	25
Turnip greens $\frac{1}{2}$ *cup cooked*	30

Fruits

Apples, baked *1 lge and 2 tbs sugar*	200
fresh *1 lge*	100
Apple sauce, sweetened $\frac{1}{2}$ *cup*	100
Apricots, canned in syrup *3 lge*	
halves and 2 tbs juice	100
dried *10 sm halves*	100
Banana *1 med, 6 in*	90
Blackberries, fresh *1 cup*	100
Cantaloupe $\frac{1}{2}$ *of a 5$\frac{1}{2}$ in melon*	50
Cherries, sweet *15 lge*	75
Cranberry sauce $\frac{1}{4}$ *cup*	100
Dates *4*	100
Figs, dried *3 small*	100
Grapefruit $\frac{1}{2}$ *medium*	50
Grapes, American or Tokay *1 bunch*	
– 22 av	75
seedless *1 bunch – 30 av*	75
Olives, green *4 med or 3 extra large*	15
Orange *1 med*	80
Peaches, canned in syrup *2 lge*	
halves and 3 tbs juice	100
fresh *1 med*	50
Pears, canned in syrup *3 halves and*	
3 tbs juice	100
fresh *1 med*	50
Pineapple, fresh *1 slice $\frac{3}{4}$ in thick*	50

	Calories
Plums, canned *2 med and 1 tbs juice*	75
fresh *2 med*	50
Prunes, dried *4 med*	100
Pumpkin *½ cup*	50
Raisins *¼ cup*	90
Raspberries, fresh *1 cup*	90
Rhubarb, stewed and sweetened *½ cup*	100
Strawberries, fresh *1 cup*	90
Tangerines *1 med*	60
Watermelon *1 round slice 6 in in diam, 1½ in thick*	190

Cakes, cookies, breads and cereals

Biscuit, *2 in in diam*	100
Breads, Boston brown *1 slice 3 in in diam ¾ in thick*	90
corn (1-egg) *2 in square*	120
cracked wheat *1 slice av*	80
dark rye *1 slice ½ in thick*	70
light rye *1 slice ½ in thick*	75
white enriched *1 slice thin*	55
wholewheat 100% *1 slice av*	75
Cake, chocolate or vanilla with no icing *1 piece 2 x 2 x 2 in*	200
chocolate or vanilla with icing *1 piece 2 x 1½ x 2 in*	200
Corn *½ cup*	70
Corn syrup *1 tbs*	75
Corn flakes *1 cup*	80
Corn meal *1 tbs uncooked*	35
Cornstarch pudding *½ cup*	200
Crackers, graham *1 square*	35
round snack-type *1 cracker 2 in in diam*	15
rye wafers *1 wafer*	25
saltines *1 cracker 2 in sq*	15
Flour, white or whole grain *1 tbs unsifted*	35
Gingerbread, hot water *2 x 2 x 2 in*	200
Hominy grits *¾ cup cooked*	100
Macaroni *¾ cup cooked*	100
Muffins, bran *1 med*	90
1-egg *1 med*	130
Noodles *¾ cup cooked*	75
Oatmeal *¾ cup cooked*	110
Pies, apple *3 in sector*	200
lemon meringue *3 in sector*	300
mincemeat *3 in sector*	300
pumpkin *3 in sector*	250
Popcorn, plain *1½ cups popped*	100
Rice *¾ cup cooked*	100
Waffles, *1 waffle 6 in in diam*	250
Wheat, flakes *¾ cup*	100
germ *1 tbs*	25
shredded *1 biscuit*	100

Miscellaneous

Almonds *12–15*	100
Cashew nuts *4–5*	100

	Calories
Chocolate, milk sweetened *1 oz*	140
fudge *1 piece 1 in sq x ¾ in thick*	100
malted milk *fountain size*	460
Gelatin, fruit flavored, dry *3 oz pkg*	330
Hickory nuts *12–15*	100
Honey *1 tbs*	100
Ice cream *½ cup*	200
Ice cream soda *fountain size*	325
Jellies and jams *1 rounded tbs*	100
Maple syrup *1 tbs*	70
Molasses *1 tbs*	70
Oil – corn, cottonseed, olive, peanut, sunflower *1 tbs*	100
Peanut butter *1 tbs*	100
Peanuts, shelled *10*	50
Pecans *6*	100
Pickles, cucumber sour and dill *10 slices 2 in in diam*	10
sweet *1 small*	10
Salad dressing, French *1 tbs*	90
mayonnaise *1 tbs*	100
Sherbert *½ cup*	120
Soup, condensed *11 oz can* mushroom	360
noodles	290
tomato	230
vegetable	200
Sugar, brown *1 tbs*	50
granulated *1 tbs*	50
powdered *1 tbs*	40
Walnuts *8*	100

Drinks

1. Alcohol

beer *8 oz*	120
gin *1½ oz*	120
rum *1½ oz*	150
whiskey *1½ oz*	150
Wines	
champagne *4 oz*	120
port *1 oz*	50
sherry *1 oz*	40
table, red or white *4 oz*	95

2. Non-alcoholic drinks

Cola, soft drinks, *6 oz bottle*	75
Ginger ale *1 cup*	85
Grapefruit juice, unsweetened *1 cup*	100
Grape juice *½ cup*	80
Prune juice *½ cup*	100
Tomato juice *1 cup*	60

9 ARE ALCOHOL AND SMOKING HEALTH HAZARDS ?

Alcohol

In moderation alcohol is a boon and a blessing, but taken in excess it is a major cause of personal unhappiness and social upheaval. It is also a considerable factor in causing organic and psychiatric illness.

Drinking too much alcohol can cause gastritis, digestive tract cancers, cirrhosis of the liver, damage to the brain and nervous system, musculoskeletal disorders and other conditions. By 'too much' I mean the regular consumption of more than three or four drinks every day.

Alcohol can also cause heart disease and this is commoner than is generally realized. It is difficult for the doctor to diagnose, particularly in the early stages, because the patient's drinking history may be the only clue to its presence. There is no specific test, such as the electrocardiogram in coronary disease, which will establish the diagnosis. Also, heart disease in the alcoholic may be dominated by his other medical and behavioural problems.

Although alcohol is not a direct cause of coronary heart disease and stroke, there is no doubt that the heavy drinker is at high risk because his habits and life-style make him prone to atherosclerosis. Obesity is common in the heavy drinker because of the high calorie content of alcohol and because, except in the most severe alcoholics, it increases the appetite.

Heavy, steady drinkers are prone to Type-4 hyperlipidaemia, one of the blood-fat disturbances mentioned earlier (page 87). This blood-fat disturbance increases the risk of atherosclerosis and in my experience in Ireland is almost confined to heavy drinkers. The blood fat quickly returns to normal when the person stops drinking. There is strong evidence that heavy drinking may cause or aggravate high blood pressure. It certainly makes effective drug treatment of high blood pressure more difficult.

Because of his environment and the people he meets, the heavy drinker is more likely to be a cigarette smoker and, if he has stopped smoking, he is more likely to start again. Nor is it likely that he takes much exercise. He is also frequently affected by personal and social stress.

This is not the place to discuss the treatment of alcoholism except to say that it is an increasingly serious problem in Western countries. Although many aspects of the treatment of obesity can be used to overcome alcoholism, specialist help will be needed. To successfully combat drinking the alcoholic will need the utmost compassion and interest from family and close friends. Physical exercise and a physical fitness programme may be very beneficial for an alcoholic, but exercise is generally not sufficiently emphasized in treatment. Leisure interests and activities may also be helpful – anything to break the vicious cycle.

The benefits of exercise are illustrated by the following case history.

M. O. is a businessman from a country town in Ireland. He had a very bad history of alcoholism with several admissions to psychiatric hospitals for treatment. He was a source of unhappiness and despair to his family and friends and his business was going downhill.

At the age of forty-eight he met a doctor who told him to start walking and to join Alcoholics Anonymous. He started walking regularly and now walks six miles briskly every day. I saw him at the age of fifty-nine and, unlike the chronic alcoholic who is characterized by muscle wasting of the shoulders, hips and thighs, he had the physique of a man of thirty to forty. A maximum-exercise electrocardiogram was consistent with the performance of a man twenty years younger and confirmed that he was as active as he stated. He has never taken a drink since. He leads a busy life at business and still takes part in A.A. affairs. He says that each day is brightened for him by the prospect of his six-mile walk.

Cigarette smoking

Cigarette smoking is the major cause of illness and premature death in modern Western society. The numerous reports from the Surgeon General of the United States and the Royal College of Physicians in London, together with the reports and recommendations issued by hundreds of other health agencies, all support this.

These reports and recommendations are based on extensive and thorough research and will be confirmed by the experience of every physician. There is no evidence available to refute the conclusions arrived at by the Surgeon General and by the Royal College of Physicians.

Coronary heart disease, stroke, vascular disease of the legs, chronic bronchitis, emphysema, respiratory failure and lung cancer are all directly caused or aggravated by smoking. Other diseases associated with smoking are cancer of the throat and bladder, duodenal ulcer, chronic catarrh, sinusitis, and dental decay.

It is not surprising, therefore, in view of the high frequency of these diseases in Western countries, that cigarette smoking is very prevalent in the West. It is also not surprising that the Consumers Consultative Committee in the United Kingdom estimates that tax revenue raised in Great Britain from tobacco tax (£1,570,000,000 or $3,140,000,000) is only about one third of the annual loss from smoking (£4,4011,500,000 or $8,8023,000,000).

In a number of medical reports my colleagues and I showed that coronary patients smoked twice as heavily as a healthy control group. The Framingham group (page 87) also identified cigarette smoking as a major factor associated with coronary disease and stroke. British research workers Doll and Hill showed that smoking doctors between thirty-five and fifty-four years were four times as liable to a heart attack as their non-smoking colleagues; other research workers have shown that a coronary attack is as much as six times greater in heavy smokers compared to non-smokers.

Irish mortality statistics clearly parallel those in other Western countries. Under the age of sixty-five years, 60 per cent of all deaths were attributed to diseases in which cigarette smoking was a major cause. It was estimated that more than 2000 of the 76000 deaths which occurred in Ireland in people aged between twenty-five and sixty-five in 1974 were the direct result of smoking.

It is therefore not surprising that many authorities say that a man who smokes and inhales twenty cigarettes a day from the age of twenty will reduce his life expectation by 20-25 per cent. Heavier smokers will have a correspondingly greater loss of life expectation. In other words, the greater the number of cigarettes you smoke and the longer you have been smoking, the greater the risk of disease. The Framingham study found that men who smoked heavily were more likely to have an acute heart attack. It is also likely that the European habit of smoking cigarettes to the end is more harmful than the North American habit of throwing away a substantial amount of the cigarette.

How does cigarette smoking cause disease?
Many people are sceptical about the numerous adverse effects of smoking. How can one agent cause so many different and unrelated diseases? This is a very reasonable question but the complex biochemical and physiological actions of smoking go a long way to explain its many effects on the body.

Respiratory disease is reasonably explained by the hot airstream and the presence of a variety of toxic and cancer-causing chemicals in the tobacco smoke. The hot airstream and the toxic substances damage the delicate inner lining of the bronchial tubes and the sensitive mechanism in the lining which is designed to get rid of waste products. This mechanism gently sweeps away harmful foreign substances, just as the rotating brush in the carpet sweeper sweeps away loose debris.

Damage to this scavenging action inevitably leads to chronic infection (catarrh and bronchitis), destruction of the delicate air sacks (emphysema) and malignant changes (lung cancer). The cancer-producing substances or carcinogens in cigarettes may also account for the higher frequency of throat cancer and of bladder cancer in smokers.

There are four important ways in which cigarette smoking causes atherosclerosis, coronary disease, stroke and vascular disease of the legs:

1. There are millions of little particles in the blood called platelets. These are damaged by nicotine and are shed in excessive numbers on to the lining of the arteries where they may act as forerunners of atherosclerotic plaques. The effect of nicotine on platelets and on their excessive deposition in the arteries has been shown by careful experimental studies.

2. Nicotine increases the tendency of blood to clot in the blood vessels. The tendency is aggravated by the presence of established atherosclerosis. This may account for the high frequency of myocardial infarction and stroke in cigarette-smoking people and for the fact that risk falls gradually when they stop smoking.

3. Nicotine stimulates the production of chemical substances called catecholamines in special glands and nervous tissue. These are normally present in the tissues but they may have an adverse effect on the heart and blood vessels if they become excessive. Catecholamines increase the work and oxygen consumption of the heart, they increase the heart rate and blood pressure, and they increase the irritability of the heart. These effects may be serious in a heart already jeopardized by atherosclerotic disease. For instance, the increased irritability of the heart may lead to serious irregularities and this may account for the higher incidence of sudden death in cigarette smokers. Nicotine also stimulates the production of another chemical substance called pitressin which may constrict coronary arteries.

4. Cigarette smokers absorb a substantial amount of carbon monoxide in the airstream. The oxygen-carrying substance in the blood known as haemoglobin has a very high affinity for this gas; in other words, if cigarette smokers inhale, as much as 15 per cent of the haemoglobin may be thrown out of action by carbon monoxide. This effect may lead to an increased production of haemoglobin and red cells and to increasing thickness or viscosity of the blood. The reduction of the oxygen-carrying and oxygen-releasing power of the haemoglobin and the increased viscosity of the blood may have a detrimental effect on circulation to the heart and to the other vital organs, particularly if the arteries are already damaged and narrowed by atherosclerosis.

The dangers of inhaling

Inhalation vastly increases the risk of disease from cigarette smoking. It allows the carcinogens to reach the lining of the lungs, the bladder and elsewhere, and both nicotine and carbon monoxide enter the bloodstream in large amounts. Pipe and cigar smokers generally do not inhale and, although they do suffer damage to the gums, teeth and sinuses, they do not have a cigarette smokers' high risk of respiratory and atherosclerotic disease. If, however, you give up cigarette smoking and take up a pipe or smoke cigars – and continue to inhale – you still place yourself at risk for cigarette diseases.

Smoking and women

There is a widespread notion that women are less vulnerable than men to the effects of smoking. I don't agree.

Women *appear* to be less vulnerable to smoking because there are fewer smokers among them, they are lighter smokers and they inhale less; but the woman who smokes one or two packs a day and who inhales deeply, as most men do, is perhaps more vulnerable than a man because of her smaller size and the consequently greater concentration of nicotine and carcinogens in the body mass (page 105). I have been impressed by the extent of atherosclerosis noted at autopsy in some pre-menopausal women who smoked heavily.

What are your chances?

As in many other medical situations, people vary a good deal in their reactions to cigarette smoking. In one person the arteries may bear the full brunt, in another the

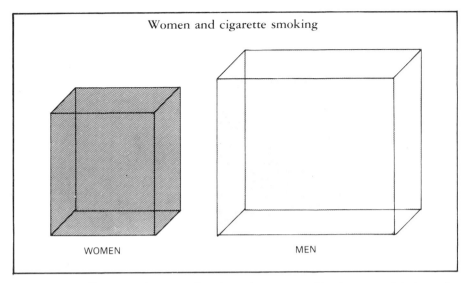

Women and cigarette smoking

WOMEN   MEN

Women may suffer a more intense effect from cigarette smoking because of their smaller body size as represented by the two boxes. The smoke inhaled by women will therefore tend to have an even more harmful effect.

lungs. In some people it is common for multiple cigarette diseases to develop. The very exceptional person may survive to a reasonably good age and have very little to show for his cigarette smoking.

There are no known tests to discover a smoker's susceptibility to disease at the early stages – and it may be too late to do so afterwards. The important point is that the inhaling cigarette smoker has a substantially reduced expectation of life in the great majority of cases and he is playing a very chancy game of roulette with his life.

The cards are also heavily stacked against the smoker's general health and physical wellbeing. Some important field studies and enquiries have shown that the habitual cigarette smoker is more liable to be sick, hospitalized, and have other problems than the non-smoker. The amount of money spent by the health services in treating cigarette diseases is greatly in excess of the tobacco tax which is collected – and this is not counting the high cost of importing tobacco leaf to countries like my own.

Has cigarette smoking any virtues?
The answer is no, and I say this having been myself a moderately heavy smoker until eighteen years ago. Claims are made that smoking is relaxing, that it has a useful, tranquillizing effect, that it is enjoyable and that it controls weight.

Let us look at these claims in turn. I agree that smoking can be relaxing and tranquillizing, but only to the person who is addicted to nicotine. A fresh cigarette will frequently relieve the withdrawal symptoms he suffers if he has not smoked for some time. These withdrawal effects are psychological and usually take the form of tension, irritability and lack of concentration. They may be associated with restlessness, skin sensations and excess salivation. The prompt relief of these symptoms by smoking is naturally interpreted as being due to the relaxing effect of the cigarette, but the non-smoker does not suffer these effects and does not require a cigarette to relax because he is already as relaxed as the satiated cigarette smoker.

There is no evidence whatever that cigarette smoking is tranquillizing. In fact its effect on the body is the exact opposite. It increases the pulse rate, blood pressure, and energy requirements, as well as the irritability of the heart. Try inhaling one or two cigarettes and check your pulse rate before and after.

Nor do I believe that cigarette smoking is really enjoyable. In my own experience the enjoyment was transient and largely caused by the relief of withdrawal symptoms. Most of my smoking, apart from the initial drag or two, seemed to be carried out in a mechanical way without any special feelings of pleasure. On the contrary, when I smoked I felt guilty and had a strong sense of personal dissatisfaction about being dependent on it.

There is a popular misconception that smokers are less likely to be overweight than non-smokers. This is wrong. Generally, there is no significant difference between the average weights of smokers and non-smokers. Confusion has arisen here because people who stop smoking often put on weight. Ex-smokers are heavier than smokers, but they are also heavier than non-smokers because they have substituted excess eating for smoking. The prevention of weight increase in ex-smokers is dealt with on pages 94–100.

In summary, no known effect of cigarette smoking has been shown to be beneficial.

What are the advantages of giving up?

If you smoke cigarettes, and manage to give it up, you will gradually and substantially reduce the risk of developing the cigarette-smoking diseases, except where there is established lung, throat and bladder cancer. This applies at any age and irrespective of how heavily and how long you have smoked. All the important field studies have shown that the risk of lung cancer and coronary disease falls over some years and that eventually the risk of the ex-smoker reaches that of the non-smoker.

It is also obvious to the physician that the symptoms of chronic bronchitis, emphysema, sinusitis and catarrh will frequently improve and will certainly not progress after giving up smoking. A duodenal ulcer will often heal in an ex-smoker, even without any other form of medical or surgical treatment, and the symptoms of vascular disease of the leg may improve or clear up completely with a greatly reduced danger of progress to gangrene and amputation.

In the course of research work at my hospital we have shown that the patient who survives a coronary attack and who stops smoking has only half the chance of a further attack and half the chance of dying compared to the patient who continues to smoke afterwards. This work has been confirmed in Sweden and America. If the inventor of coronary artery surgery could achieve these results he would have become a Nobel prize winner long ago!

After giving up smoking, you will also have healthier gums and teeth, a better sense of smell and taste, less hoarseness and a stronger voice. Not only will you feel healthier, but you will save money and feel a sense of pride at having given it up.

How to give up smoking

The key to success is good motivation and the key to good motivation is to be fully aware of the facts about smoking. You must be informed about the health hazards and the illusory benefits of smoking, and be aware that the withdrawal effects associated with stopping are entirely psychological. You may find it helpful to receive guidance about weight control and techniques of reducing or eliminating the withdrawal effects.

Reading this book might help you but you may also require the assistance of a doctor and a dietitian. A doctor who has clear convictions about the harmful effects of smoking and who is interested in your problem will help you achieve success.

Not many people are aware of the real health hazards of smoking and when they are informed of these personally by an authoritative person, such as a doctor, they will often stop. The better informed and the more strongly motivated the person, the easier it is to stop and the less severe and prolonged the withdrawal symptoms. Many well-motivated heavy smokers have expressed surprise to me that stopping was so easy and so free from unpleasant side-effects.

The easiest way to stop smoking is to do it instantly and with the intention of never smoking again. Some people stop gradually and may try using various tricks and proprietary aids but they are usually less successful, perhaps because they are less determined to give up. A gradual reduction in smoking may help, but it is easy to backslide if you have a pack of cigarettes on hand. Success must come from conviction. Of course some people find that cigarette smoking gives them up rather than the other way round; they lose all desire to smoke. This sometimes happens to pregnant women, for example, but you cannot count on that bonus.

If you are unable to give up smoking immediately (and this applies to some well-motivated people), you can often fortify yourself by reading regularly about the subject and by occasional conversations with your doctor or another ex-smoker. Try reminding yourself about the money you are saving. All these suggestions should help you succeed.

A substantial reduction in the number of cigarettes smoked will, of course, reduce the risk of the cigarette diseases. For this reason the person who is unwilling to give up, or who wishes to do so gradually, may find the following advice helpful.
1. Smoke a low-tar, low-nicotine cigarette. Information about the tar and nicotine content of cigarettes is available from heart and cancer foundations and from government health agencies. It is also clearly marked on every packet of cigarettes.
2. Smoke less of each cigarette and progressively leave more. Gradually reduce the frequency and depth of inhaling.
3. Set out daily non-smoking periods for yourself. Arrange non-smoking locations such as the car, your bedroom, mealtimes and in the presence of your children. Never offer or accept a cigarette. Substitute pipe or cigar smoking for cigarettes but do not inhale.

Side-effects of giving up smoking

Some people worry about putting on weight after giving up. This occurs because they eat more and they tend to substitute food for an after-dinner cigarette. For a long time this cigarette has provided the reflex to stop eating and it is now no longer available. You may also find yourself eating sweets and other high-energy foods between meals. Obesity is a less serious risk factor than cigarette smoking, but is still undesirable, particularly if you have angina and coronary heart disease.

Every effort should be made to avoid putting on weight and provided you are reasonably self-disciplined about it you should have no problem. The idea is to get rid of one addiction without acquiring another.

Try finishing a meal with a low-calorie food such as raw vegetables or fruit and, if you must eat between meals, stay with the low-calorie foods. Chewing-gum may also help. Regular and adequate physical exercise will help to keep your weight down. It will also help to improve your motivation and relieve the general withdrawal effects.

Former smokers who suffer from chronic cough, breathlessness and wheezing, because of bronchitis and catarrh, may find that the symptoms do not improve. They may actually worsen for a month or two after stopping. This is because the catarrh continues to form for a while and you no longer have a cigarette to make you cough and clear the air passages. With a little patience the catarrh dimishes, the cough disappears, your breathing improves and you no longer find yourself wheezing and spluttering – in short, you attain a new freedom to breathe.

Some people develop feelings of boredom and depression and may complain of insomnia when they stop smoking. These are temporary conditions. It is important to keep mentally and physically occupied. Physical exercise is a real help, particularly when aimed at enjoyment and fitness. In some cases of depression or tension a doctor may help by prescribing a tranquillizer or depression-reducing drug. While I avoid drugs if I can, there is no doubt that some people can be helped over the acute withdrawal period by a daytime tranquillizer or night-time sedative.

How to stay off cigarettes
Make a resolution – never smoke the first cigarette!

When you give up smoking you will gradually lose the craving for a cigarette. You will also forget how addictive the habit is and how difficult it was to stop. Every now and then the ex-smoker feels a brief return of the craving, particularly during convivial and social occasions. On such occasions the foolhardy may yield, mistakenly believing that he is cured of the addiction. That one cigarette may shatter morale with disastrous results.

Remember, *never smoke the first cigarette*. If you faithfully stick to this resolution you need not worry about the rest.

With full knowledge of, and insight into, the smoking habit, very few people who stop will start again. Apart from the benefits to health and fitness, you will invariably feel satisfied with your achievement.

10 HIGH BLOOD PRESSURE

Hypertension, or high blood pressure, is a major cause of ill-health and premature death. While not more important than cigarette smoking in Western countries, hypertension is the dominant cause of ill-health in other countries such as Japan where high blood-pressure levels may be related to diet and particularly to a high salt intake. A few, mostly primitive, societies do not suffer from high blood pressure.

What is blood pressure?

Blood pressure is the pressure existing inside the arteries which is responsible for maintaining the circulation. The pressure itself is maintained by the continuous output of blood from the heart and by the resistance created by the small narrow arteries in the tissues which will close up further if, for any reason, the blood pressure is required to rise. These arteries act like a partly-closed sluice gate and have an important function, not only in maintaining blood pressure but also in directing the flow of blood to the parts of the body that are most in need of it; for example, the muscles during exercise and the stomach during digestion. It is like an electric power-supply grid which can change the amount and distribution of electricity at short notice.

Normal blood pressure varies, depending on the phase of activity of the heart. It is highest during heart contraction (systole) when the volume of blood in the arteries increases suddenly. It is lowest at the end of heart relaxation (diastole) when the volume of blood reaches its lowest ebb. These are called the systolic and diastolic blood-pressure levels. Both are routinely measured by simple clinical means and the unit of measurement used internationally is the millimetre of mercury (mmhg).

Normal blood pressure is generally around 120 mmhg systolic and 80 mmhg diastolic. In fact blood pressure varies very much between individuals and may be normally lower than 100/60 or as high as 140/90. It is very difficult to define a dividing line between normal and abnormal levels. A blood pressure of 140/90 is often taken as an arbitrary dividing line if this level is constantly maintained or exceeded at each examination. In evaluating a person's blood pressure a number of factors might be taken into account. For instance, a blood pressure of 140/90 is much less significant in a sixty-year-old compared to a twenty-year-old person.

There is also considerable variation in a person's blood pressure level from one moment to another. Blood pressure is influenced by many physiological, emotional and physical factors, and this accounts for the frequent changes in blood-pressure levels. It may be at its lowest point during sleep and at its highest during fright, anger or during an emotional upset.

Blood pressure is measured by the sphygmomanometer. This is an inflatable cuff which encircles the arm and which is connected to a mercury manometer or measuring device. Air is pumped into the cuff until sufficient pressure is exerted to block the flow of blood in the arm arteries. The operator allows air to escape slowly from the cuff while listening with a stethoscope placed over the artery at the elbow. As soon as the pressure falls sufficiently to allow blood to start flowing again, there will be a sharp sound over the artery which the operator will hear. The point at which the first sound is recorded is the systolic blood pressure.

As the pressure in the cuff is further reduced to the point where there is no interference with the flow of blood, the sound in the artery disappears. The pressure reading on the manometer at this point represents the diastolic blood pressure.

With practice, it is possible to make a fairly accurate measurement of the systolic and diastolic blood pressures without using a stethoscope. The systolic pressure is identified by the first appearance of a sharp knocking in the artery within the arm. At the diastolic pressure this knocking disappears. This simpler method is adequate if you check your own blood pressure regularly.

What is high blood pressure?

This is blood pressure which is permanently higher than normal: that is, above 140/90. It is divided into two main sub-groups. Secondary hypertension is caused by diseases of the kidneys, adrenal glands and blockage of the main blood vessel or aorta. These cases are relatively rare nowadays, but are most common in young people and are important because indentification of the cause and its removal may improve or cure the high blood pressure.

The great majority of cases of high blood pressure, particularly in older people, are classified as primary or essential hypertension. Secondary hypertension is relatively rare in Western countries. Essential hypertension is very common.

The results of blood-pressure screening of the Irish adult male population carried out by the Irish Heart Foundation about eight years ago illustrate the high frequency of raised blood-pressure levels. It was also found that identification and treatment of blood pressure by doctors was unsatisfactory.

Five per cent of all males aged between twenty-five and sixty-five years had diastolic blood-pressure readings of 110 or more and another 14 per cent had diastolic figures between 95 and 109. In other words, nearly 20 per cent of the adult male population had mild or more severe high blood pressure.

Only 30 per cent of these had had their high blood pressure noted by a doctor and, of these, again, only 30 per cent were considered to be receiving adequate treatment. In other words, only about 12 per cent, or one in eight, of the population with high blood pressure was having satisfactory treatment. The same frequency of hypertension has been reported from the United States, the United Kingdom and other Western countries. With community programmes and public education the situation is now improving.

While blood pressure tends to increase with age in Western countries it should not be accepted as a normal phenomenon. A perfectly healthy person's mean blood pressure should not increase with age; the increasing blood pressure in the population reflects the increasing number of hypertensives in the older age groups.

There is no evidence that high blood pressure is a new disease but it is probable that secondary hypertension is much less frequent nowadays because of the decline in the prevalence of kidney trouble. On the other hand, essential hypertension may be commoner because of social, cultural and dietary changes, but we have insufficient evidence to prove this.

What can happen when you have high blood pressure?

Raised blood pressure, even if it is very high, does not cause symptoms in the absence of complications. You may notice a vague or unusual degree of fatigue, but the presence of more severe symptoms such as headaches, dizziness, breathlessness, or swelling of the ankles, indicates the early development of complications or the presence of anxiety and nervous symptoms.

High blood pressure is important because of the common and often lethal complications. The frequency of these complications in the untreated person depends directly on the severity of the blood pressure rise and its duration.

The important complications of high blood pressure are: stroke, coronary heart disease, heart failure and kidney failure.

Stroke may be due to the rupture of an artery in the brain because of high internal pressure. This is more likely to occur if the artery is already diseased by atherosclerosis, very commonly found among high blood-pressure patients.

Most cases of stroke in high blood-pressure patients are due to narrowing and blocking of atherosclerotic arteries to the brain, leading to temporary or permanent reduction or cutting off of blood supply with consequent localized brain damage.

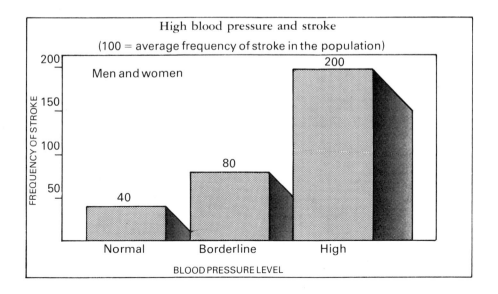

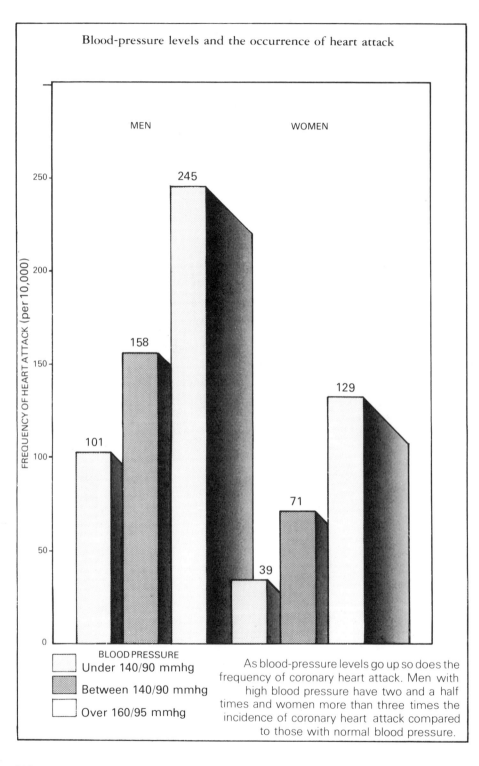

Blood-pressure levels and the occurrence of heart attack

MEN

WOMEN

FREQUENCY OF HEART ATTACK (per 10,000)

245

158

101

129

71

39

BLOOD PRESSURE
Under 140/90 mmhg

Between 140/90 mmhg

Over 160/95 mmhg

As blood-pressure levels go up so does the frequency of coronary heart attack. Men with high blood pressure have two and a half times and women more than three times the incidence of coronary heart attack compared to those with normal blood pressure.

The incidence of stroke, and particularly stroke from cerebral haemorrhage, is falling rapidly in Western countries, almost certainly because of the improved diagnosis and treatment of high blood pressure.

Coronary heart disease Blood pressure is one of three principal risk factors for angina and heart attack because of its association with atherosclerosis. The longer hypertension is present and the higher its level, the greater the risk (page 112).

Doctors are still not sure whether treatment of high blood pressure will affect the incidence of coronary heart disease. In the United States and Scandinavia, however, high blood pressure is better controlled nowadays and coronary heart disease is less common than it used to be. It seems reasonable to link the two, although we can't yet show a direct connection.

Disease of the leg arteries, as described on page 37, is also common in hypertensives.

Heart failure The increasing stress of high, uncontrolled blood pressure may eventually lead to rather sudden and possibly lethal failure of the left ventricle of the heart. Fortunately, with modern treatment of hypertension and with improved identification of sufferers, this complication is becoming a rarity.

Kidney failure may occur when blood pressure accelerates. In this condition, called malignant hypertension, there is a progressive rise in blood pressure to lethal levels which may interfere with, or destroy, the kidneys. Fortunately, this complication is also preventable with modern drug treatment.

The risk of the atherosclerotic diseases: stroke, heart attack and disease of the leg arteries will be aggravated by the presence of other important risk factors such as cigarette smoking, abnormal blood fats and poorly controlled diabetes. For instance, if you have a mild to moderately raised blood pressure you have about twice the risk of coronary heart attack compared to a person with normal blood pressure. If the hypertensive person also smokes a pack of cigarettes or more per day, his risk of heart attack may increase to ten times or more than that of the non-smoking person with normal blood pressure. So don't take risks!

If you have uncomplicated high blood pressure you will not need elaborate tests or investigations before treatment is started. Complicated and severe cases and young patients with secondary hypertension may need to be examined by a specialist and this may require a stay in hospital. The main objects of investigation are to establish the cause and severity of the high blood pressure, to evaluate the condition of the arteries and vital organs, to decide the proper treatment and to identify other risk factors. For instance, a blood cholesterol test should be made in all cases as part of the initial investigation.

Can high blood pressure be controlled or cured?
In a few people, particularly among the young, high blood pressure caused by kidney, adrenal gland or disease of the aorta and kidney arteries can be cured. There

is no immediate and permanent cure, however, for cases of essential hypertension or hypertension associated with chronic kidney damage.

The patient with essential hypertension is like the diabetic. In both cases, the patient can control the disease himself with modern treatment which will greatly reduce the risks and complications. If he stops treatment, the condition will recur sooner or later. The following case history is typical of many:

B.D. had a life-insurance examination in 1961 when he was thirty-eight years old. His blood pressure was raised at the time and the life-insurance premium was substantially increased. The high blood pressure was again noted in 1964 during a routine medical examination. Despite these findings, neither he nor his doctor took any action to treat the condition.

In 1968 he noticed shortness of breath when walking and climbing stairs. This symptom became noticeably worse over a period of about six weeks and culminated in a severe attack of breathlessness and gasping which awoke him from sleep one night. He was rushed to hospital where a diagnosis of acute heart failure due to severe and untreated high blood pressure was made. Emergency treatment restored the function of his heart and during the following ten days his blood pressure was brought under complete control with appropriate drugs.

Ten years later, B.D., who is now fifty-five, leads a normal life and has fully controlled high blood pressure. He checks his own blood pressure about once a week and he sees his doctor every three months. Occasional adjustments in the dose of the drugs are required, but his blood pressure has been virtually normal for ten years and he has no evidence of heart failure nor of heart disease. His case is typical of the benefits to be gained by sticking to treatment.

If you are hypertensive it is clearly important to have a thorough knowledge of the principles of your treatment. You need a good rapport with your doctor. Play a permanent part in your own treatment and you can lead a life-style in keeping with a long, active life.

Treatment of high blood pressure
The first step in treatment is to decide if it is necessary. This can only be done by your doctor. In doubtful or borderline cases drug treatment may not be necessary but your blood pressure will need to be checked regularly every three to six months and you will be advised about weight, exercise, smoking and other habits.

If there is a cause for the high blood pressure it must be sought and removed, and if your hypertension is well established you will almost certainly require drug treatment. There have been great advances in the drug control of high blood pressure over the past twenty-five years and practically every case of essential hypertension can be controlled by drugs. Only the physician can decide the correct drug treatment and it may take time, and trial and error, before treatment is established.

Although the doctor will decide your treatment, you should take a close interest in his advice and you should be aware of certain important aspects of the treatment:
1. Stick to the dose and combination of drugs prescribed by your doctor. Do not stop

treatment without his knowledge and advice. Drug treatment does *not* cure blood pressure, it controls it and treatment may be necessary over many years, or even permanently.

2. Learn the side-effects that may be associated with the drug. Recognize these effects and how to manage them.

You can assist your own treatment, just as diabetics do, by learning how to take blood pressure regularly and you should keep a diary of blood-pressure figures, weight, drug dosage and other useful information. Some people, by manipulating drug dosage under the close supervision of their doctor, can keep blood pressure at normal levels and yet avoid significant side-effects. Some doctors believe that regular blood-pressure measurement by patients may cause anxiety and excessive introspection, but I have yet to find this in well-informed people.

Doctors are often asked if high blood pressure should be treated after the development of a heart attack or stroke. The answer here is a definite yes. Proper treatment of high blood pressure will almost certainly reduce the risk of a furthur attack and will also reduce the chances of other complications.

Salt and high blood pressure

Most people eat far too much salt and this may be dangerous if you have high blood pressure. Although not proved, there is strong evidence from international field studies to suggest that any community which, as a whole, eats a great deal of salt is also liable to suffer from high blood pressure.

It is believed that an intake of approx. $\frac{1}{10}$ oz (2–4 g) of sodium chloride or salt is the daily need of an adult under normal climatic conditions. In fact the average intake in most communities is in excess of $\frac{1}{3}$ oz (10 g), while some people who are heavy salt eaters may eat up to $\frac{2}{3}$ oz (20 g) per day. In countries, such as Japan and South Korea, where high bood pressure is common, heavy salt eating is associated with preserving fish and meat in salt. Also the blood pressure of American school-children has been shown to be highest in areas with a large salt content in the drinking water.

I believe that no free salt should be consumed with food, and extremely salty food, like salted peanuts, should be avoided. Parents should keep an eye on their children's eating habits since free salt eating is often a habit acquired during childhood. Taking the salt cellar off the table is the easiest way to cut out the habitual adding of salt to food.

If you stop using excessive salt you will miss it for a while but within a short time you will have forgotten about it and be left with the true taste of food – as I have found. There are plenty of salt substitutes if you need added taste. Mustard, lemon juice, vinegar, spices and proprietary salt substitutes are only a few.

Many doctors advise people with high blood pressure to avoid salt and salty foods. We have no real evidence that it helps once the high blood pressure has been established but it may reduce the tendency to aggravation of the blood pressure and to complications. I certainly think that, if you have early or borderline high blood pressure, you may avoid raising it by being strict about your salt intake.

As an example of recent important trends in the community control of blood pressure I think it is worth mentioning our experience in Ireland, a country of just over three million people. In co-operation with the Department of Health and with our community doctors and nurses, the Irish Heart Foundation has established seventy hypertension screening clinics throughout the country. Adults are invited to come for a blood-pressure check at these clinics and, if their blood pressure is high, the patient is advised to attend his or her family doctor for further examination and for treatment if necessary.

This experiment in community blood-pressure control has been running for two years and is an excellent and successful example of the benefits of co-operation between the medical and nursing professions, the health authorities and the community at large. It is receiving widespread public support and appreciation with more than 3000 people already sent to their doctor for investigation and treatment of high blood pressure.

It is obvious that we need more efficient screening to identify hidden high blood pressure and to offer treatment before any damage is caused to arteries or vital organs. The present situation is very hopeful in that better identification and treatment of high blood pressure in countries like the United States has dramatically reduced death rates from hypertensive heart failure and kidney failure and has greatly reduced the incidence of stroke. The improving trends in coronary disease mortality in some countries may be related to better blood-pressure treatment. There is no doubt that the continuing improvement in professional and public education on blood-pressure control will greatly reduce the hazards of this widespread disease.

11 WHAT OTHER FACTORS AFFECT HEART DISEASE AND STROKE?

Stress

Does stress cause disease? In particular, does it cause heart disease? Despite a great deal of research, we do not really know. It is hard to define what we mean by stress, although I think of it as 'the physical and emotional responses to a situation where the person is psychologically or emotionally poorly adapted to his environment'. This is a rather wide definition and certainly one which is difficult to measure.

It is claimed that stress may be commoner nowadays as a result of the increasing dynamism and activity of urban life. This claim needs examination on two scores. Firstly, I doubt if there is any proof that stress is commoner nowadays, although I do not deny the possibility. Secondly, if stress is more common, what elements in modern life have been responsible? Is it because we have to work harder and because life is more competitive and more complicated, or, more likely, because we do less physical work and now have a vacuum created by increased leisure time?

Other factors, such as the dislocation of family and marital life, disturbed personal relationships, and a rapidly changing sense of values in a consumer society should also be considered.

There may be a certain personality type who is more prone to heart attack than others. He is sometimes classified as a 'Type A' and the extreme case is described as a fist-clenching, desk-banging, dynamic executive type who is constantly fighting time schedules and attempting to maintain climbing graphs. In contrast, the more passive and less ambitious 'Type B' is considered to be less liable to heart trouble (page 118).

Type A may produce more catecholamines, or the 'drive' hormones, than other people and perhaps this indirectly causes atherosclerosis through increased blood pressure and through the increased mobilization of fatty acids in the blood. The Type A may smoke and drink more, although research workers who support the Type A concept say that its influence is independent of the three main risk factors for coronary disease: cigarette smoking, hypertension and abnormal blood fats.

Certainly, the catecholamines may cause increased heart work and an increased heart rate, and may induce irritability of the heart, which in a person with jeopardized coronary circulation may lead to fatal irregularities and sudden death.

I am not totally convinced that a Type A personality is more liable to athero-sclerosis and heart disease. As a clinical cardiologist, in close contact with hundreds of cases of coronary disease every year, I have not found a dominance of any personality type. It may be that a valid appreciation of personality type is too subtle for the practising physician and requires complicated psychological tests for its

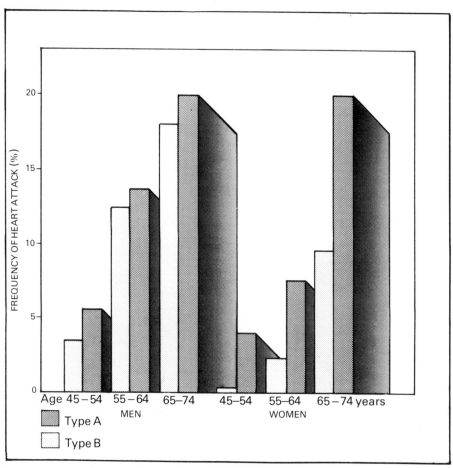

The occurrence of coronary heart disease among men and women of different age groups is here divided into personality types A and B, type A being characteristically more tense and type B taking life more gently.

identification, but is is worth pointing out that coronary disease is now substantially less common in the executive and professional classes than in the blue- and white-collar classes in such 'dynamic' communities as the United Kingdom and the United States.

There is evidence, however, that emotional stress may precipitate an acute heart attack in a coronary-prone individual. Patients with established coronary heart disease are generally advised to avoid exciting and tension-packed occasions, such as football matches and racing, in which they may increase the irritability of the heart muscle and may precipitate an attack.

There is also some evidence that a myocardial infarction is more likely to occur in a coronary-prone person after some unusual or disturbing life event such as divorce, a change in occupation, a bereavement or loss of work. Again, this type of association is very difficult to measure and to establish.

The possible association between long-term stress and high blood pressure may be more important. We know little about the causes of essential hypertension but we know that it is very common in modern society and almost certainly has a number of causes. It is impossible for the practising physician to avoid the impression that emotional upset, tension, anxiety and chronic personal conflicts are important in aggravating, and perhaps in initiating, high blood pressure. We know that trans-cendental meditation can reduce the level of persistent high blood pressure and a number of surveys have shown that the average blood pressure of people on vacation is lower than it is in their normal working and domestic environment. If you have high blood pressure you should take every step to eliminate unnecessary stress from your life, even if you have to make difficult or drastic changes to do so.

There is some evidence that stress and prolonged anxiety may cause blood cholesterol to rise but, again, we are not sure about this either. It has been shown that cholesterol levels are higher in students before examinations than afterwards. Chronic stress may increase dependence on alcohol and cigarette smoking and thus, indirectly, contribute to an unhealthy life-style and to a propensity to heart disease.

Stress, therefore, militates against good health and positive living. Every effort should be made to harmonize our personal, domestic and business lives. You may need help from friends, family, physician or psychologist, but most of all you need a good insight into your own personality and relationships and a proper sense of values.

More than anything else I would recommend the virtues of exercise, physical fitness, recreation and sport, and creative leisure-time occupations and hobbies to sustain interests and to put the problems and stresses of life in their proper perspective.

Age

Coronary heart disease and other results of atherosclerosis become more frequent with increasing age. Coronary disease is probably highest between sixty and seventy years. Atherosclerosis is not part of the natural ageing process and there is no reason why a healthy man of eighty should not have clear and atheroma-free arteries. Arteries do normally become harder and more rigid with age but this is caused by an accumulation of fibrous tissue and chalk in the middle or medial coats of the arteries. This gives the old person's arteries a hard, prominent look but from the health point of view this is of no significance.

Atherosclerosis is always abnormal, no matter at what age it occurs. The reason it is commoner in older people is because they have had a longer time to accumulate it.

Family history

It is not uncommon to find that more than one person in a family gets a coronary heart attack. Sometimes whole families seem to suffer, occasionally developing the disease at an early age. Some people therefore think that if you are born into a family with a history of heart disease you must be more likely to have a heart attack irrespective of the way you live.

I am not convinced that heredity, as a primary risk factor, is important. And this is a hopeful view for those with a strong family history of the disease because our origin and our parents are things we can do nothing about. Nobody has yet come up with convincing evidence to show that your parents' history of heart disease or stroke has a direct bearing on your own.

Many of the well-known risk factors, however, tend to be commoner in some families than others. Your family may have a tendency to high blood pressure, abnormal blood fats or obesity. Smoking, eating and other habits tend to be shared by members of the same family. If one member of your family has heart disease you need to look carefully at any risk factors you may have, such as smoking. If there are no risk factors, or you get rid of them, your family history need cause you no concern.

Women

In affluent Western communities and in people under fifty years old, coronary disease is about four times more common in men than in women. Men also die more often from coronary disease. After the age of fifty, and as the older age groups are reached, women suffer more heart attacks and, eventually, have as many as men.

Since younger men are more liable to heart disease than younger women, many people believe that men are more vulnerable to atherosclerosis and its consequences, either because of a special constitutional predilection or because women are protected by some attribute peculiar to their sex. It is believed, for instance, that women, before the menopause, are unlikely to develop atherosclerosis because of oestrogen protection. (Oestrogen is a female sex hormone which is present in abundance before the menopause.) There is not much evidence to support these views.

There are other, and more plausible, reasons why women suffer less from coronary disease up to the age of sixty. A research study reported from my hospital in the American heart journal, *Circulation*, confirms that hypertension, hyperlipidaemia and cigarette smoking dominate among women coronary patients, as they do among men. The reason coronary disease may be less common among younger women is that the intensity of these three factors is considerably less among them.

Fewer women smoke and they smoke considerably less than men. They are also less likely to inhale deeply. The average daily consumption of cigarettes by men in the United Kingdom is ten per day compared to about three per day by women.

Our own research studies (page 88), and reports from elsewhere, have shown that male cholesterol levels in the healthy population begin to rise in the late twenties or early thirties and reach a peak about the mid-fifties. Female cholesterol levels remain at a relatively low level until the mid-forties and are significantly lower than the male levels. The female levels begin to rise significantly about the time of the menopause and this rise will continue up to and beyond sixty years, where the levels will first reach and then pass the male level. Cholesterol in women before the menopause tends to be carried in the high-density lipoproteins, a form which is certainly less harmful and may even be protective. The lower cholesterol levels of younger women may be due to some glandular effect, but equally it may be due to differences in the eating habits and life-styles of men and women.

High blood pressure has also been shown, in various field surveys, to be significantly lower in pre-menopausal women, but to rise and to exceed the male blood pressure level in the late fifties. Stroke is also commoner in younger men than women although the differences here are less than in coronary heart disease.

The important point about women is that those with coronary disease have the same risk factor background as men. Women who are exposed to one or more of these factors are at high risk, even before the menopause, and, if you are a woman, you should be as conscious as men of the need to avoid unnecesary risk.

The contraceptive pill can be a cause of heart attack and stroke, but for all practical purposes it is only important in older women and in those with other risk factors such as cigarette smoking. It is also best avoided if you have a previous history of blood clotting. If you use a contraceptive pill, and are at all doubtful about it, you should discuss it with your doctor.

Drinking water

People living in areas with hard or lime-rich water tend to have a lower mortality from heart disease than those who live in soft-water areas. In fact, mortality from all causes tends to be higher in soft-water areas, which suggests that the quality of water does not influence the death rate from heart disease. It is much more likely that mortality is related to the fact that the higher social classes, with lowest mortality, tend to live in hard-water areas. For all practical purposes you need not worry whether you drink soft or hard water – at least so far as the atherosclerotic diseases are concerned.

Occupation and accidents

In some countries, and in certain states in the United States, it is legally accepted that heart attacks may result from particular occupations. In such cases substantial damages and disability pensions are sometimes paid. I know of no convincing evidence that any occupation, whether it is considered stressful, heavy or leading to 'overwork', can be the cause of atherosclerosis and heart attack. I suspect that a coronary event or stroke is often attributed to work or worry because of an understandable wish to find a virtuous reason for human misfortune. A reference to the victim's unhealthy life-style or habits would just add to his troubles. Apart from an increase in coronary disease in association with certain chemical industries, I know of no scientific or acceptable evidence to link occupation with heart disease and stroke.

Heart attacks are also frequently attributed to accidents, and particularly to motor accidents. In my view these claims are usually made on insufficient evidence. There are relatively few well-documented cases of myocardial infarction where the attack could be attributed to direct or indirect injury to the chest. Occasionally, direct injury to the chest may lead to coronary obstruction and myocardial infarction but usually only if the person has well-established disease in the arteries. In other cases, after a severe injury with a profound drop in blood pressure, the circulation in the coronary arteries may be impaired in a person with atherosclerosis and he may suffer an infarction at that time.

If you suffer a heart attack at, or immediately after, an accident there may well be a connection. If it occurs some days or weeks later it is very unlikely to be caused by the accident. Apart from direct bruising and tearing of the heart, heart damage is a very remote possibility in anyone who suffers an accident and who has had a healthy heart beforehand.

A lesson worth learning

Sometimes heart disease can be a blessing in disguise, as the following case history reveals.

P.S.D. comes from a professional family. He is intelligent but not academically minded and so refused to go on to higher education. Instead he joined a small electrical maintenance firm and qualified as an electrician. Soon afterwards he took over the small business and his active personality, combined with an exceptional capacity for work, led to rapid expansion.

He had played Rugby and tennis at school but soon all his time was taken up with his work and business contacts. These contacts led to business luncheons and evening meetings in pubs and restaurants. He became a regular heavy drinker and believed that eating and drinking with his clients was necessary for the success of his business.

He smoked two packs of cigarettes a day, his life became more stressed and more frenetic and he saw less and less of his wife and three children.

By the time he was thirty-eight he was about 60lb (27 kg) overweight. He took no exercise and he was wheezy and breathless on exertion. He was irritable with his family and life really had few joys for him, except the satisfaction of being the head of a successful electrical outfit.

At thirty-eight he felt a bad chest-pain while driving his car. It lasted for about ten minutes. He thought it was indigestion and that it was caused by the considerable amount of drink he had had the night before. Two days later he got a longer attack at home. His wife became alarmed and called a doctor and he found himself in hospital with a confirmed diagnosis of coronary insufficiency. The doctors noted his excess weight and chronic bronchitis. Tests showed that his general health was affected by his drinking, obesity and sedentary life. He had abnormal blood fats and poor ability to burn up sugar. He had a high uric-acid reading, which indicates a tendency to arthritis and gout. His drinking, excessive and unbalanced eating, smoking and lack of activity were predictably destroying the arteries, lungs and other vital tissues.

The rest of the story is instructive. No heart muscle damage occurred but clearly he had underlying atherosclerosis. Seven days later, when he was leaving hospital, he had clear instructions about a new and heathy life-style. That was five years ago.

P.S.D. is now forty-three. He realizes that prolonged business luncheons with too much food and alcohol play no part in achieving success. The turnover of his business has increased fivefold since his illness; he delegates more work but is still firmly at the helm. He takes two holidays a year, one with his wife and children, and the other with his wife. He sails every Saturday in season and goes orienteering in the mountains with his family every Sunday. He is an enthusiastic runner and plays squash. He does not smoke and I am certain he will never smoke again. He drinks socially but is no longer dependent on alcohol.

P.S.D. enjoys life in every way; he seldom has a spare moment, but is under no stress. His chronic bronchitis has cleared up and a recent maximum-stress test shows excellent circulation to the heart muscles. His sugar metabolism is normal, as is his weight, and his blood fats have also returned to normal.

He eats the same food as his wife and children – a balanced diet without excessive amounts of animal food, fat and refined sugar. He takes no free salt but eats low-calorie foods such as salads, raw and cooked vegetables and fruit. He admits that his life has taken on a new and meaningful dimension.

Do not think that this case history is an unusual one. The preventive-minded doctor can dig out dozens of these case histories from his file.

ACKNOWLEDGEMENTS

I am grateful for vauable assistance received from Mrs Vivien Reid; Commandant Finn Monahan and the Staff of th Irish Heart Foundation; the staff of the Coronary Heart Research Unit at St Vincent's Hospital; Mrs Herma Boyle and Commandant Maurice Cogan of University College, Dublin.

I want to thank Gussie Mehigan and Barton Kilcoyne whose interest in exercise and physical fitness had an important impact on my own attitudes. I am particularly grateful to my colleague, Dr Noel Hickey, whose commitment to heart-disease prevention has always been a great inspiration to me. Miss Nancy Gorgan, my secretary at St Vincent's Hospital, prepared all the manuscripts. Her patience and good humour made my task relatively easy.

John Rutt provided a great deal of advice and patient guidance for the indoor and outdoor exercise chapters — especially in organizing and directing the photographic sessions. Rosemary Pettit edited the manuscript. Martin and Ruth Dunitz were helpful and patient publishers.

I am most grateful to Professor John Goodwin who wrote the foreword and made very helpful criticisms, and to Michelle Corbiére for the warmth of her hospitality whilst I was writing this book in Provence.

The publishers would like to thank: Lennart Nilsson and ICI Pharmaceuticals for the photographs on page 16; Pictor International for the photographs on pages 4 and 57; the World Health Organization; the Metropolitan Life Insurance Co., New York; Dr William Kannel; Professor Ancel Keys; Professor Jerry Stamler; Dr Geoffrey Dean; Dr Alicia Radic; Dr I. Hjermann; Professor Joossens and Robert Eagle, editor of *Pain Topics*.

Thanks also to all those who modelled, including: Jon Bannenberg, Albert Parry, Yvonne Smith and Julia Drake; to Slick Willies and Brodie Sports for the loan of tracksuits.

Charts were prepared using research material derived from the following:
Framingham study, pages 36, 86, 111, 112, 118
Metropolitan Life Insurance Co., New York, pages 93, 97–9
St Vincent's Hospital, Dublin, page 90
Study by author and colleagues, pages 85, 89
World Health Organization, page 25
Canadian Medical Association Journal and the World Health Organization, page 95

124

INDEX

acupuncture 89
acute coronary insufficiency 30, 31, 122
acute heart attack: *see* myocardial
    infarction
after-care 28, 34, 35, 42
ageing 11, 23, 39, 40, 110-11
alcohol 43, 89, 94, 101-2, 122, 123
angina 24, 26-30, 43, 108, 113
aorta 19, 23, 110, 113
arteries *16*, 17, 19-21, 34-5, 104, 109,
    110, 111, 113, 116, 119, 122, 123
    see also angina; atherosclerosis; leg
    vessel disease
arteriogram, coronary 24, 27, 29, 35
arthritis 15, 38, 39, 64, 66, 68, 72,
    123
atherosclerosis 13, 22-4, 26, 27, 29,
    34, 35, 37, 39, 101, 103, 104, 111,
    117, 119, 120

blood 17-21, 24, 39, 103, 104
    fats 23, 35, 37, 39, 84-5, 87-91, 94,
        101, 113
    see also cholesterol
    pressure 14, 23, 26-7, 34, 38, 39,
        90, 94, 101, 104, 106, 109-16,
        119, 120-1
    sugar 37, 39
bypass operation 29, 36-7

calisthenics 41, 42, 55, 59-62, 63-83
cancer 4, 101, 102, 103, 106
cardio-respiratory system 39-40, 41
case histories 15, 28, 102, 114, 122-3
catecholamines 103-4, 117
cholesterol 22, 23, 24, 36, 39, 84-91,

113, 119, 120-21
circulatory system 17-21, *18*, *20*, 21
clotting 22, 33, 40, 103
contraceptive pill 121
coronary care units 29, 31-2
coronary occlusion; coronary
    thrombosis: *see* myocardial infarction
cycling 26, 41, 56-8, *57*

depression 38-9, 94, 108
diabetes 23, 38, 94
diet 14, 42, 84, 85, 88-9, *190*, 114-15
    against obesity 24, 94, 96, 108
    see also cholesterol; obesity; salt
disc trouble 15, 38, 59.
Doll and Hill 102-3
drugs 29, 34, 36, 38, 91, 100, 101,
    108, 113, 114, 155
Dublin hospital patients 33-4, 87,
    89-90, 106

electrocardiogram (ECG) 27, 31, 42
embolism 22, 34, 37
    see also plaques
exercise and fitness 24, 26, 28, 33, 34,
    37, 38-83, 89, 100, 101, 108, 119

family history and disease 23, 119-20
food *see* diet; obesity
Framingham study 87, 102

gardening 33, 40, 41, 100
golf 41, 62

'hardening of the arteries' 22
health education 13, 14, 15